Radiation Therapy for Head and Neck Cancers

Murat Beyzadeoglu • Gokhan Ozyigit
Ugur Selek

Editors

Radiation Therapy for Head and Neck Cancers

A Case-Based Review

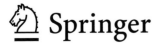 Springer

Editors
Murat Beyzadeoglu, MD
Professor and Chairman
Department of Radiation Oncology
Gulhane Military Medical School
Ankara
Turkey

Ugur Selek, MD
Professor and Chairman
Department of Radiation Oncology
Koc University, Faculty of Medicine
Istanbul
Turkey

Gokhan Ozyigit, MD
Professor and Chairman
Department of Radiation Oncology
Hacettepe University
Faculty of Medicine
Ankara
Turkey

ISBN 978-3-319-10412-6   ISBN 978-3-319-10413-3   (eBook)
DOI 10.1007/978-3-319-10413-3
Springer Cham Heidelberg New York Dordrecht London

Library of Congress Control Number: 2014954994

Printed on acid-free paper

Springer is part of Springer Science+Business Media (www.springer.com)

*Dedicated to the memory of Professor
Kie Kian Ang, MD, PhD (1950–2013)*

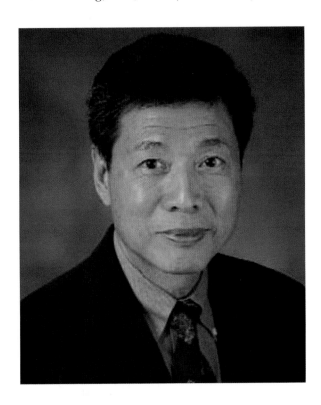

Preface

Head and neck region is a challenging region of the body, containing critical parts associated with basic physiological functions including respiration, nutrition, and expression. Debilitating consequences may occur as a result of head and neck cancers depending on location, size, and spread pattern of the tumors. Structural disfiguration and functional impairments may considerably compromise social integration and quality of life. Therefore, optimal management of head and neck cancer patients requires a multidisciplinary team approach with the endpoint of functional survival.

The intent of writing "Radiation Therapy for Head and Neck Cancers – A Case-Based Review" was to provide a structured, comprehensive Head & Neck book to furnish the practicing healthcare providers with a contemporary evidence-based management guide to fulfill the goal of having "cured" but functionally unimpaired patients.

Each clinical chapter includes several head and neck cancer cases for the demonstration of target volume delineation and intensity-modulated radiotherapy treatment planning. Several cross-sectional slices of both contouring and planning images are included in order to give a more complete picture for each clinical case. Three chapters cover the general management issues, systemic therapies, and complications of head & neck radiotherapy. Furthermore, important clinical trials are also provided for evidence-based management in each head & neck subsite. In summary, readers can find every practical and theoretical aspect of modern radiotherapy approach from consultation phase to treatment delivery stage in "Radiation Therapy for Head and Neck Cancers – A Case-Based Review".

We extend our most sincere gratitude to our patients teaching us invaluable lessons more than we can learn from books while they are suffering from physical and mental pain in their combat with cancer.

Ankara, Turkey, 2014   Murat Beyzadeoglu, MD
Ankara, Turkey, 2014   Gokhan Ozyigit, MD
Istanbul, Turkey, 2014   Ugur Selek, MD

Acknowledgements

The editors are indebted to Ute Heilman, Corinna Schäfer, and Wilma McHugh from Springer DE and Kalpana Venkatramani and Mahalakshmi SathishBabu from SPi for their assistance in preparing *Radiation Therapy for Head and Neck Cancers: A Case-Based Review*.

We extend our most sincere gratitude to Professor Hayati Bilgic, the dean of Gulhane Military Medical School, and to our colleagues and friends at Gulhane Military Medical School, Faculty of Medicine at Hacettepe University, Koc University, and Baskent University, as well as to our families for their understanding as we worked to meet our publication deadlines.

Contents

Contributors

Sercan Aksoy, MD Associate Professor, Department of Medical Oncology, Hacettepe University, Cancer Institute, Sihhiye, Ankara, Turkey

Murat Beyzadeoglu, MD Professor and Chairman, Department of Radiation Oncology, Gulhane Military Medical School, Etlik, Ankara, Turkey

Yasemin Bolukbasi, MD Associate Professor, Department of Radiation Oncology, MD Anderson Radiation Treatment Center, American Hospital, Nisantasi, Istanbul, Turkey

Mustafa Cengiz, MD Professor, Department of Radiation Oncology, Hacettepe University, Faculty of Medicine, Sihhiye, Ankara, Turkey

Ferrat Dincoglan, MD Assistant Professor, Department of Radiation Oncology, Gulhane Military Medical School, Etlik, Ankara, Turkey

Melis Gultekin, MD Assistant Professor, Department of Radiation Oncology, Hacettepe University, Faculty of Medicine, Sihhiye, Ankara, Turkey

Pervin Hurmuz, MD Assistant Professor, Department of Radiation Oncology, Hacettepe University, Faculty of Medicine, Sihhiye, Ankara, Turkey

Gokhan Ozyigit, MD Professor and Chairman, Department of Radiation Oncology, Hacettepe University, Faculty of Medicine, Sihhiye, Ankara, Turkey

Cem Parlak, MD Assistant Professor, Department of Radiation Oncology, Baskent University, Faculty of Medicine, Adana, Turkey

Omer Sager, MD Assistant Professor, Department of Radiation Oncology, Gulhane Military Medical School, Etlik, Ankara, Turkey

Yucel Saglam, MSc Radiotherapy Physicist, Department of Radiation Oncology, MD Anderson Radiation Treatment Center, American Hospital, Nisantasi, Istanbul, Turkey

Sezin Yuce Sari, MD Instructor, Department of Radiation Oncology, Hacettepe University, Faculty of Medicine, Sihhiye, Ankara, Turkey

Ugur Selek, MD Professor and Chairman, Department of Radiation Oncology, Koc University, Faculty of Medicine, Nisantasi, Istanbul, Turkey

Department of Radiation Oncology, University of Texas MD Anderson Cancer Center, Houston, TX, USA

Mehmet Ali Sendur, MD Assistant Professor, Department of Medical Oncology, Yıldırım Beyazıt University, Faculty of Medicine, Ankara, Turkey

Erkan Topkan, MD Associate Professor and Chairman, Department of Radiation Oncology, Baskent University, Faculty of Medicine, Adana, Turkey

Gozde Yazici, MD Associate Professor, Department of Radiation Oncology, Hacettepe University, Faculty of Medicine, Sihhiye, Ankara, Turkey

Berna Akkus Yildirim, MD Instructor, Department of Radiation Oncology, Baskent University, Faculty of Medicine, Adana, Turkey

General Concepts in Head and Neck Radiotherapy

1

Murat Beyzadeoglu, Omer Sager, and Ferrat Dincoglan

Overview

Although accounting for approximately 4 % of all carcinomas, an important group of tumors both numerically and epidemiologically arise in the head and neck region with diverging disease courses that may pose formidable challenges in therapeutic management. This relatively small region of the body contains critical parts associated with basic physiologic functions including respiration, nutrition, and expression. Debilitating consequences may occur as a result of head and neck cancers depending on location, size, and spread pattern of the tumors. Structural disfiguration and functional impairments may considerably compromise social integration and quality of life. Moreover, treatment of the disease may induce additional mutilations and dysfunctions with the potential to further aggravate quality-of-life impairment.

A multidisciplinary team approach is needed for optimal management of patients with head and neck cancers, and mortality should not simply be regarded as the sole measure for survival with the understanding that these cancers may induce substantial morbidity. Maintaining functionality and decreasing the structural deformities are critical aspects of management. In this context, decisions to achieve maximal cure and functionality with minimal morbidity, and maintaining the capability to salvage recurrent disease should be addressed at the very outset. Initial assessment and designation of individualized treatment algorithm should involve active participation from the multidisciplinary team of experts. Likewise, prevention and management of treatment-related sequelae warrant the involvement of specialists with

M. Beyzadeoglu, MD (✉) • O. Sager, MD • F. Dincoglan, MD
Department of Radiation Oncology, Gulhane Military Medical School,
Etlik, Ankara, Turkey
e-mail: mbeyzadeoglu@yahoo.com

© Springer International Publishing Switzerland 2015
M. Beyzadeoglu et al. (eds.), *Radiation Therapy for Head and Neck Cancers:
A Case-Based Review*, DOI 10.1007/978-3-319-10413-3_1

expertise in their field. Treatment of patients within this wide spectrum of the disease may be satisfactory but also disappointing since treatment-induced morbidity may be hazardous even when substantial regression of large tumors is achieved. Patients with acute treatment-related morbidity are usually hardly manageable in the course of their treatment due to poor nutrition and performance status. With the recent technological advances in radiation oncology discipline, factors of maintaining the quality of life, preservation of structure, functionality, and cosmesis have become indispensable management goals to be considered. Improved imaging capabilities may allow earlier diagnosis which may translate into preserved voice and swallowing functions. Optimal selection of treatment modality based on meticulous staging workup is necessary. In this aspect, detailed knowledge of fundamental oncological principles along with thorough patient evaluation is mandatory. Interdisciplinary collaboration of radiation oncologists, surgical oncologists, and medical oncologists is crucial with the inevitable support of dental oncologists, maxillofacial prosthodontists, pathologists, radiologists, nutritionists, reconstructive surgeons, neurosurgeons, oncology nurses, psychiatrists, social workers, physical medicine and rehabilitation physicians, speech and swallowing therapists, neurology service, and other health care personnel involved in management and rehabilitation of head and neck cancer patients. Coordination among the disciplines may offer the best chance of cure with optimal functional and cosmetic outcomes. Nevertheless, the patient's active involvement is another important aspect of successful management. Whichever individualized treatment algorithm is recommended, the patient may prefer a therapeutic approach that offers better functional or cosmetic outcomes at the cost of a lower probability of tumor control. That is why active participation of the patients in decision making process is important.

1   Natural History

Head and neck cancers mostly follow an orderly and predictable spread pattern. Approximately two thirds of the patients have locally advanced disease at presentation. A tendency towards local or regional spread is common in head and neck cancers. Regional involvement is frequently concerned with the primary tumor's anatomic location and extent. Despite the increased risk of hematogenous spread in the presence of enlargement and extracapsular extension of the involved neck nodes, distant metastasis constitutes an infrequent pattern of failure, which allows potential cure by optimal management strategies. Nevertheless, head and neck tumor sites of the nasopharynx and hypopharynx have a relatively higher likelihood for distant spread. The most common site of distant failure is the lungs

Table 1.1 Head and neck lymphatics

Level	Lymphatics
Ia	Submental lymphatics
Ib	Submandibular lymphatics
II	Upper jugular lymph nodes
III	Middle jugular lymph nodes
IV	Lower jugular lymph nodes (transverse cervical)
V	Spinal accessory chain lymph nodes (posterior triangle)
VI	Prelaryngeal, pretracheal, paratracheal lymph nodes

followed by the bones, mediastinal lymphatics, liver, and brain secondaries. However, atypical distant involvement of cutaneous and subcutaneous tissues may occur in patients with radical neck dissection or previous radiotherapy. Due to the risk of nerve invasion for some head and neck tumors, particularly for parotid cancers, nerve traces should meticulously be considered in the treatment planning process.

Head and neck tumors accounting for approximately 4 % of cancers may present with diverse natural histories that make their management more complex. They are named according to their locations and subsites in the head and neck region [1]. Head and neck cancers are usually seen in patients over 40 years of age, while salivary gland and nasopharyngeal cancers may occur at earlier ages. Women are more frequently affected compared to men. Certain types are more commonly observed in certain geographic locations (e.g., nasopharyngeal cancer in Far East Asia). Smoking, tobacco, and alcohol are considered as major risk factors for head and neck cancers. Chewing tobacco and tobacco-like substances have been associated with increased risk of oral cavity cancers [2].

Other risk factors for head and neck cancers include genetic predisposition, previous head or neck cancer, history of cancer in the immediate family members, exposure to ionizing radiation as well as to sun (ultraviolet radiation), nutritional disorders and habits, vitamin deficiencies, iron-deficiency anemia, poor oral hygiene, use of inappropriate prostheses, chronic infections, gastroesophageal reflux, and specific viral infections (EBV, HPV) [3, 4]. Head and neck cancers may occur simultaneously or metachronously in multiple locations in the same individual [5]. Exposure to radiation may occur through several ways, such as prior radiotherapy directed at the head and neck area or radioactive contamination from nuclear reactor accidents (e.g., Chernobyl) or nuclear weapons (e.g., Hiroshima and Nagasaki). Human papillomavirus infection (HPV) has been shown to have a role in the development of particularly oropharyngeal cancers [6, 7].

There is a rich lymphatic network in the head and neck area (Table 1.1). Level I lymphatics include the submental and submandibular area. Levels II, III, and IV include upper internal jugular, middle internal jugular, and lower internal jugular lymph nodes, respectively. Level V includes posterior triangle, and level VI includes prelaryngeal, pretracheal, and paratracheal lymph nodes.

This lymphatic network is divided into sublevels for purposes of neck dissection or radiotherapy (Fig. 1.1).

Fig. 1.1 Lymphatic levels of the neck for head and neck cancers

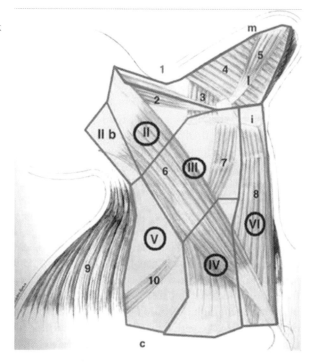

Over 30 % of all head–neck cancer cases show clinical lymph node positivity (Table 1.2) [1, 9]:
Pharyngeal wall cancer: 50 %
Pyriform sinus cancer: 49 %
Supraglottic laryngeal cancer: 39 %
Head–neck cancers with clinical neck lymph node (−) but pathological lymph node (+) (Table 1.2) [9]:
Pyriform sinus cancer: 59 %
Pharyngeal wall cancer: 37 %
Tongue cancer: 33 %
Supraglottic laryngeal cancer: 26 %
Floor of mouth cancer: 21 %
Glottic laryngeal cancer: 15 %

Table 1.2 Lymphatic involvement ratios in various head–neck cancers (%) [1, 8]

Region	Level I		Level II		Level III		Level IV		Level V		RPLN	
	N–	N+	N–	N+	N–	N+	N–	N+	N–	N+	N–	N+
Nasopharynx											40	86
Tongue	14	39	19	73	16	27	3	11	0	0	–	–
Base of tongue	4	19	30	89	22	22	7	10	0	18	0	6
Retromolar trigone	25	38	19	84	6	25	5	10	1	4	–	–
Tonsil	0	8	19	74	14	31	9	14	5	12	4	12
Pharyngeal wall	0	11	9	84	18	72	0	40	0	20	16	21
Pyriform sinus	0	2	15	77	8	57	0	23	0	22	0	9
Supraglottic larynx	6	2	18	70	18	48	9	17	2	16	0	4
Glottic larynx	0	9	21	42	29	71	7	24	7	2	–	

RPLN retropharyngeal lymph nodes

2   Pathology

Most cancers arising from the upper aerodigestive mucosa are squamous cell carcinomas (SCC) or one of its variants including lymphoepithelioma, spindle cell carcinoma, verrucous carcinoma, and undifferentiated carcinoma. Adenocarcinoma, mucoepidermoid carcinoma, and adenoid cystic carcinoma are seen in the major salivary glands including the parotid, submandibular and sublingual glands, as well as the minor salivary glands. Merkel cell carcinoma most frequently arises on the head and neck skin and is among the cutaneous neuroendocrine neoplasms. Merkel cell tumors follow an aggressive disease course with common locoregional and distant failure. Lymphomas, solitary plasmocytomas, soft tissue sarcomas, melanomas, and other malignant and benign neoplasms represent the remaining cases.

3   Workup

A meticulous physical examination including the palpation of the head and neck lymph node regions, direct or indirect visualization of the primary site by mirror, or fiberoptiscopic examination is an important part of initial patient assessment. Imaging studies include computed tomography (CT) and/or magnetic resonance imaging (MRI) of the head and neck region and X-ray examinations of the skull, sinuses, and soft tissue. Barium swallow may be suggested for symptomatic patients, along with chest radiograph and bone scan to exclude metastatic disease. Integrated positron emission tomography (PET)/CT imaging may assist in precise definition of locoregional disease and distant metastases. It may also aid in locating occult tumors in the setting of an unknown primary and may be beneficial for detecting recurrent disease after treatment. Viral titers may be elevated in some patients, anti-Epstein–Barr virus antibody titers may be used to assist in the diagnosis of nasopharyngeal cancers in some cases. Laryngoscopy, bronchoscopy, and esophagoscopy may be considered in the setting of suspected synchronous aerodigestive primary.

Staging of head and neck cancers is mostly based on clinical diagnostic information about the tumor size, extension, and presence of involved lymph nodes. Decision making for adjuvant treatment warrants accurate surgical–pathological classification.

4   Radiation Therapy Planning and Treatment Procedure

Radiation therapy process for head and neck cancers generally include the following steps:

- Positioning for treatment, immobilization, and imaging for treatment planning
- Contouring of treatment volumes and organs at risk (OARs)
- Dose prescription
- Forward planning (3-dimensional conformal radiation therapy, 3DCRT) or inverse planning (intensity-modulated radiation therapy, IMRT)
- Plan assessment and improvement
- Implementation of plan and treatment verification

5   Patient Preparation and Immobilization

Positioning of the patient for treatment may depend on the specific cancer type being treated and the objectives of the treating physician concerning the tumor volume and normal tissue sparing. Patient lies supine in the majority of cases with the neck extended and the head on headrest. Surgical scars and palpable nodes may be wired. The patient should be immobile during therapy. Movements may cause changes in the treatment area and increase side effects, thus affecting treatment success. The patient should be positioned in the most comfortable, easily reproducible way suitable for the irradiated region of interest.

Optimum immobilization is a major component of radiotherapy management in head and neck cancers. The importance of setup reproducibility is becoming more important with the need for tighter margins and steep dose gradients in the modern radiotherapy era.

Thermoplastic face mask is frequently used for immobilization of patients with head and neck cancers (Fig. 1.2).

Such a mask should not only be tight but also there should be no space between the patient's skin and the mask. The mask should be checked during every setup

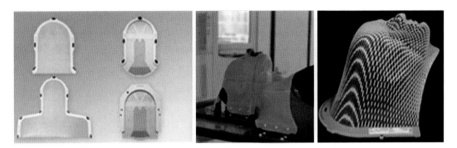

Fig. 1.2 Thermoplastic mask

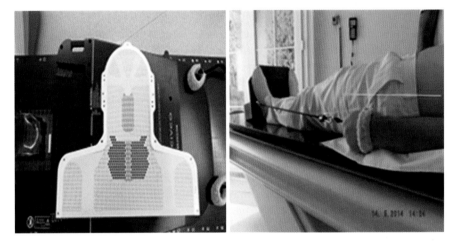

Fig. 1.3 Immobilization mask and shoulder retractor (Courtesy of Gulhane Military Medical Academy)

procedure for tightness or looseness (due to edema or weight loss) and should be remade adaptively if necessary.

Immobilization of patients for irradiation of the head and neck region is usually provided by means of a support under the head with aquaplast cast for facial fixation (with or without shoulder inclusion), both attached to a baseplate on top of the treatment couch. Shoulder retractors may be used to remove shoulders from the treatment field to allow appropriate low-neck irradiation (Fig. 1.3).

Bite-block is frequently used in oral tongue radiation treatments. A small hole can be made in the mask if a bite-block or nasogastric tube is being used. An effective tongue blade with a cork attached to one end may displace the tongue out of the treatment volume, and mucosal sparing of the hard palate may also be achieved by displacing the palate.

Inadequate immobilization may result in inaccuracies. Erroneous alignment of treatment fields causes interfraction errors. Intrafraction errors may occur if the patients and/or tumor volumes move during treatment delivery as a consequence of incorrect immobilization or physiologic activity. Accounting for these uncertainties in the treatment planning and delivery processes poses a formidable challenge and is an area of active investigation.

6   Simulation

Simulation is defined as radiotherapy field determination using a diagnostic X-ray machine (conventional or CT based) with similar physical and geometrical features to the actual teletherapy machine. The patient is immobilized before simulation, and then the tumor is localized either in a direct scopy X-ray machine or in serial CT slices. The simulation can be done by CT, MRI, or rarely by PET/CT.

Determination of the patient's treatment position and construction of the immobilization device are typically performed in a dedicated radiation therapy CT-simulator room including a diagnostic quality CT scanner, laser patient positioning/marking system, virtual simulation 3D treatment planning software, and various digital display systems for viewing the digitally reconstructed radiographs (DRRs) [10–12].

The mask and other required equipment are made on the day of CT simulation by the radiotherapist, under the supervision of the radiation oncologist, for the patient who is to receive radiotherapy (Fig. 1.4).

The patient is sent to the nurse for an IV route before CT simulation if an IV contrast material is to be used. Then, the patient is positioned on the CT couch, and the mask, knee support, alpha cradle, or any other similar device is fitted on the CT couch if required. The lasers are turned on, and they are positioned at the midline according to the region of interest. Reference points are determined by radiopaque markers located at the cross sections of the lasers (Fig. 1.5).

Reference points are predetermined locations for each region of the body. There are three reference points: one is craniocaudal, and the others are on the right and left lateral sides.

Contrast material is given intravenously by the nurse, if required. Adequate measures should be taken for any possible anaphylactic reactions. Any required adjustments are performed by the CT technician in the CT command room (Fig. 1.6).

The region of interest (that for which serial CT slices are to be taken) is determined by the radiation oncologist. The slice thickness is also determined. All of these data are transferred to the CT computer. After the region of interest has been verified on screen, serial slices are taken.

Initially, CT topograms are generated and reviewed before the acquisition of the planning scan to verify patient alignment, and relevant adjustments are performed if required. Radiopaque markers may be placed both on the aquaplast and at three levels on the patient's skin. These serve as the fiducial marks which aid in relevant coordinate transformation. Treatment planning CT is acquired using a slice thickness of 2–5 mm and should typically include the entire supraclavicular region with an approximate number of 50–200 slices totally. In some circumstances, however,

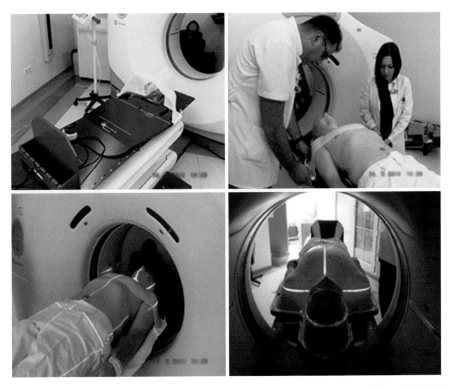

Fig. 1.4 Immobilization and simulation procedures (Courtesy of Gulhane Military Medical Academy)

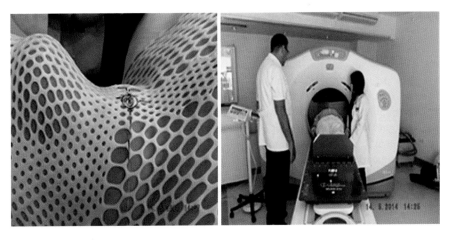

Fig. 1.5 Fiducial marks and patient simulation

Fig. 1.6 A command room for computerized tomography simulator

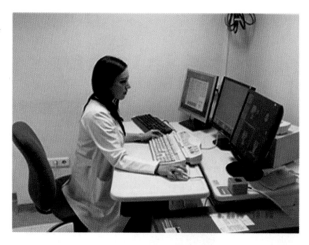

slice thicknesses of 1 mm may be required for contouring of fairly small volumes like the optic nerves and chiasm. Treatment volumes and relevant critical structures are outlined on consecutive slices to generate the structure set. Planning CT data allows for the generation of a three-dimensional anatomic model of the patient and provides electron density information to be used in the calculation of three-dimensional dose distribution. Administration of intravenous contrast may improve the visualization of the parotids and may assist in contouring of primary tumor and nodal disease.

7   Treatment Planning

IMRT warrants precise definition of treatment volumes and OARs. Uncertainties in the definition of tumor extensions and target volumes may directly affect treatment outcomes. The treatment planning process typically starts with contouring of treatment volumes and OARs. The recent report ICRU 83 has updated the definitions of volumes [13] with the consideration that volumes are more relevant in IMRT. Three types of tissue is included in the volumes which are (a) malignant lesion, (b) otherwise normal tissue close to the tumor which is already or likely to be infiltrated by microscopic disease, and (c) more distant normal tissue and organs [13].

Contouring of CTV requires clinical experience. An important difference in IMRT applications includes the quantitative definition of treatment volumes and critical structures. The use of complementary information from multimodality imaging may facilitate this process by providing additional data about disease extent. Also, contouring atlases may assist in delineation (Fig. 1.7).

Normal structures typically included in the structure set are the spinal cord, brainstem, parotid glands, skin, mandible, oral cavity, submandibular glands, lacrimal glands, glottis, brachial plexus, optic pathway, retina, lenses, lips, and inner and middle ears.

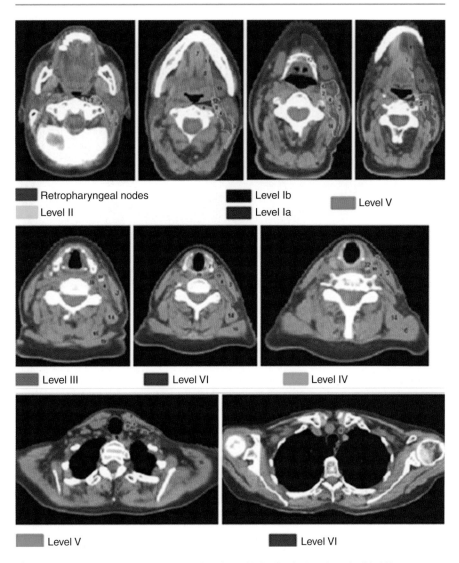

Fig. 1.7 Consensus guidelines for the delineation of N0 (elective) neck nodes [1, 14]

Physical and imaging findings are used in the delineation of gross primary tumor, nodal disease, and high-risk subclinical disease. Contouring of treatment volumes and OARs on the volumetric planning CT images is typically done by the radiation oncologist and the medical dosimetrist working as a team. OARs with distinct boundaries such as the skin and lungs may be autocontoured and slightly edited if needed. However, delineation of some critical structures such as the brachial plexus requires active participation of the radiation oncologist in the contouring process. The planning CT data set is typically transferred to treatment planning system (TPS) via the computer network.

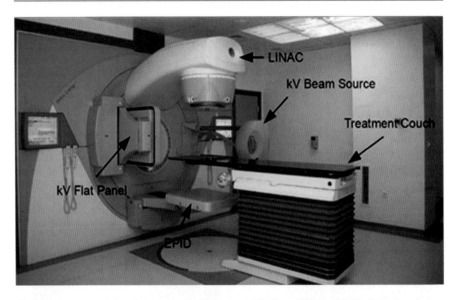

Fig. 1.8 Image-guided radiotherapy unit (Courtesy of Gulhane Military Medical Academy)

Contemporary anatomic imaging modalities including CT and MRI allow for constructing three-dimensional patient anatomy. Structure sets including target volumes and organs at risk (OAR) are defined in consecutive image slices frequently by using additional information from complementary functional imaging such as positron emission tomography (PET). Improved imaging technologies aid in the precise identification of target volumes and their relationship with critical normal tissues. With the availability of computer-controlled multileaf collimator (MLC) systems and development of linear accelerators integrated with advanced volumetric imaging systems, accurate modification and positioning of dose distributions have been possible (Fig. 1.8).

Intensity-modulated radiation therapy (IMRT) has emerged as a major technical innovation in the modern era. As a highly developed form of 3DCRT, IMRT provides a highly conformal dose distribution around the target through the use of nonuniform beam intensities. This is achieved through using either static or dynamic segments. The isodose distribution can then be matched closely to the target by modulating the intensity of each subsegment [1, 8]. IMRT may optimize the therapeutic ratio with improved control of dose distributions by manipulation of beam intensities and the incorporation of image-guided techniques for precise target contouring and treatment delivery.

This most sophisticated form of three-dimensional conformal radiation therapy (3DCRT) has been shown to be useful for decreasing long-term morbidity in nasopharyngeal, oropharyngeal, and paranasal sinus cancers through reducing doses to critical organs including the salivary glands, temporal lobes, and auditory and optic structures without compromising locoregional control [15–21]. Superior dose distributions and reduced critical organ doses in IMRT are achieved by using beamlets of nonuniform intensities delivering nonuniform dose to the target to achieve the desired dose conformality. Thus, an important advantage of IMRT is its capability to achieve higher conformality of dose distributions than those provided by 3DCRT with uniform intensity of beams. Head and neck cancers frequently need concave-shaped treatment volumes to improve sparing of critical structures (the spinal cord, brainstem, etc.) in close vicinity. Even 3DCRT may fail to achieve these fluence dose distributions, but IMRT using inverse planning algorithm in which the desired clinical and dosimetric objectives are stated mathematically may provide excellent dose distributions closely following the shapes and boundaries of target and relevant OARs in 3 dimensions. Another advantage of IMRT is that it allows easier production of nonuniform absorbed dose distributions if needed for treatment of a volume within another defined volume which is also called concomitant boost or simultaneous integrated boost [22–24]. Clearly, this precise treatment technique is more unforgiving for positioning and motion uncertainties, which warrants its use in conjunction with image-guided radiation therapy (IGRT). IGRT may be defined as the integration of various radiological and functional imaging techniques in order to perform high-precision RT. The main aims are to reduce setup and internal margins and to account for target volume changes during RT, such as tumor volume decrease or weight loss (adaptive RT). IGRT is not an IMRT technique; however, it enables various RT techniques, including IMRT, to be delivered more accurately.

Radiation treatment is indicated for most head and neck cancers since tumors in this region are frequently not amenable to optimal surgery. Nevertheless, optimal management may only be achieved through an interdisciplinary approach including experts. Patient preferences, age, performance status, comorbidities, daily habits and lifestyle, and occupation should be taken into consideration.

Preoperative radiation therapy is favored if optimal surgical resection is not feasible initially. With the use of preoperative RT, some unresectable tumors may convert to a resectable status. Also, oxygenation is better in the preoperative setting compared to postoperative setting which makes the application of preoperative RT more favorable when the tumor is more radiosensitive. Preoperative RT may also reduce the extent of normal tissue resection.

Indications of postoperative RT include close or positive surgical margins, tumor extension into soft tissues of the neck or skin, bone or cartilage invasion, perineural and/or vascular space invasion, the presence of neck nodes ≥ 3 cm, involvement in multiple lymph node levels, or nodal extracapsular extension.

Treatment is quite complex for head and neck cancers. Treatment decisions should be based on specific disease site, stage, and pathologic findings. Surgery and radiation therapy (RT) are the major curative treatment modalities for head and neck cancers. Chemotherapy only may not be curative and however is included in combined modality management to exploit the advantages of synergistic effect, particularly for stages III or IV disease. Stage I–II disease may be managed with surgery or RT only. Choice of treatment is dependent on several factors including the location and extension of the primary tumor, differentiation of cancer and cell type, morphologic tumor characteristics, status of nodal disease, the presence or absence of distant metastasis, probability of speech or swallowing function preservation, and patient preference.

Stage at the time of diagnosis is a predictor of survival and aids in decision making for management of head and neck cancers. While stages I or II disease usually define a relatively smaller primary tumor without lymphatic spread, stages III and IV disease include larger tumors with regional nodal involvement and/or invasion of underlying structures. Distant metastasis at presentation is infrequent.

Pre- and Post-radiotherapy Management Pearls

Serious temporary or permanent functional handicaps may occur as a result of high-dose radiation exposure. Appropriate prophylactic pretreatment measures may prevent or reduce the severity of these potential morbidities.

Dental prophylaxis is warranted when the mandible or the salivary glands are at the risk of receiving high-dose irradiation. Assessment of the patient by an expert dentist with special interest in head and neck cancers and the effect of RT on the oral cavity should be performed. Restoration of carious or broken teeth should be performed by a dentist or oral surgeon. Non-restorable teeth should be extracted, and RT should be initiated at least 2 weeks after extraction to allow for adequate healing. Full mouth extraction of restorable teeth should be avoided since it is considered detrimental due to increased risk of oral trauma and osteoradionecrosis. The patients should be instructed to maintain dental hygiene in the course of treatment and afterwards.

Nutritional support before, during, and after treatment is needed for all patients with head and neck cancers. Patients should be instructed to avoid using alcohol and tobacco. The use of hot and acidic fluids during RT should be discouraged. Calorie supplements and blenderized diets should be suggested for maintaining adequate nutrition of the patient.

Patients with head and neck cancers should be encouraged to maintain close contact with the treating physician for meticulous and continued follow-up. Since an overwhelming majority of recurrences occur within the first 2 years of treatment, close and meticulous follow-up is of utmost importance particularly during this time interval. Frequent follow-up of the patient should be considered for dealing with treatment-related morbidities, detecting recurrent disease and second primary cancers at an early stage.

References

1. Beyzadeoglu M, Ozyigit G, Ebruli C (2010) Basic radiation oncology, 1st edn. Springer, Berlin
2. Wannenmacher M, Debus J, Wenz F (2006) Strahlentherapie. Springer, Berlin, pp 344–345
3. Mellin H, Friesland S, Lewensohn R et al (2000) Human papillomavirus (HPV) DNA in tonsillar cancer: clinical correlates, risk of relapse, and survival. Int J Cancer 89:300–304
4. Mendenhall WM, Logan HL (2009) Human papillomavirus and head and neck cancer. Am J Clin Oncol 32:535–539
5. Schwartz LH, Ozsahin M, Xhang GN et al (1994) Synchronous and metachronous head and neck carcinomas. Cancer 74:1933–1938

6. D'Souza G, Kreimer AR, Viscidi R et al (2007) Case–control study of human papillomavirus and oropharyngeal cancer. N Engl J Med 356:1944–1956
7. Gillison ML, Koch WM, Capone RB et al (2000) Evidence for a causal association between human papillomavirus and a subset of head and neck cancers. J Natl Cancer Inst 92:709–720
8. Chao KS, Wippold FJ, Ozyigit G et al (2002) Determination and delineation of nodal target volumes for head-and-neck cancer based on patterns of failure in patients receiving definitive and postoperative IMRT. Int J Radiat Oncol Biol Phys 53(5):1174–1184
9. Lindberg RD (1972) Distribution of cervical lymph node metastases from squamous cell carcinoma of the upper respiratory and digestive tracts. Cancer 29:1446
10. Halperin EC, Wazer DE, Perez CA, Brady LW (2013) Perez and Brady's principles and practice of radiation oncology, 6th edn. Lippincott Williams & Wilkins, Philadelphia, p 207
11. Mutic S, Palta JR, Butker EK et al (2003) Quality assurance for computed-tomography simulators and the computed-tomography-simulation process: report of the AAPM Radiation Therapy Committee Task Group No. 66. Med Phys 30:2762–2792
12. Perez CA, Purdy JA, Harms WB et al (1994) Design of a fully integrated three-dimensional computed tomography simulator and preliminary clinical evaluation. Int J Radiat Oncol Biol Phys 30:887–897
13. ICRU Report 83: prescribing, recording, and reporting intensity modulated photon beam therapy (IMRT) (2010) J ICRU 10
14. www.rtog.org CT-based delineation of lymph node levels in the N0 neck: DAHANCA, EORTC, GORTEC, RTOG consensus guidelines. Accessed Jan 2009
15. Chi A, Nguyen NP, Tse W et al (2013) Intensity modulated radiotherapy for sinonasal malignancies with a focus on optic pathway preservation. J Hematol Oncol 6:4
16. Al-Mamgani A, Van Rooij P, Tans L et al (2013) Toxicity and outcome of intensity-modulated radiotherapy versus 3-dimensional conformal radiotherapy for oropharyngeal cancer: a matched-pair analysis. Technol Cancer Res Treat 12:123–130
17. Kam MKM, Leung S-F, Zee B et al (2007) Prospective randomized study of intensity-modulated radiotherapy on salivary gland function in early-stage nasopharyngeal carcinoma patients. J Clin Oncol 25:4873–4879
18. De Arruda FF, Zhung J, Narayana A et al (2006) Intensity modulated radiation therapy (IMRT) for treatment of oropharyngeal carcinoma: the MSKCC experience. Int J Radiat Oncol Biol Phys 64:363–373
19. Chao KS, Ozyigit G, Blanco AI et al (2004) Intensity-modulated radiation therapy for oropharyngeal carcinoma: impact of tumor volume. Int J Radiat Oncol Biol Phys 59:43–50
20. Lee N, Xia P, Quivey JM et al (2002) Intensity-modulated radiotherapy in the treatment of nasopharyngeal carcinoma: an update of the UCSF experience. Int J Radiat Oncol Biol Phys 53:12–22
21. Eisbruch A, Kim HM, Terrell JE et al (2001) Xerostomia and its predictors following parotid-sparing irradiation of head and neck cancer. Int J Radiat Oncol Biol Phys 50:695–704
22. Franceschini D, Paiar F, Meattini I et al (2013) Simultaneous integrated boost-intensity-modulated radiotherapy in head and neck cancer. Laryngoscope 123:E97–E103
23. Wu B, McNutt T, Zahurak M et al (2012) Fully automated simultaneous integrated boosted-intensity modulated radiation therapy treatment planning is feasible for head-and-neck cancer: a prospective clinical study. Int J Radiat Oncol Biol Phys 84:e647–e653
24. Weeks KJ, Arora VR, Leopold KA et al (1994) Clinical use of a concomitant boost technique using a gypsum compensator. Int J Radiat Oncol Biol Phys 30:693–698

Current Systemic Therapy Options for Head and Neck Cancers

2

Mehmet Ali Nahit Sendur and Sercan Aksoy

Abbreviations

CF	Cisplatin-fluorouracil
EORTC	European Organization for Research and Treatment Cancer
GETTEC	French Groupe d'Etude des Tumeurs de la Tête et du Cou trial
GORTEC	French Head and Neck Oncology Radiotherapy Group
OS	Overall survival
PFS	Progression-free survival
TCF	Docetaxel-cisplatin-fluorouracil
VALCSG	The Department of Veterans Affairs Laryngeal Cancer Study Group

Overview

Head and neck cancers comprise a heterogeneous group of malignancies which have an unsatisfactory prognosis despite intensive local treatment. Recurrences of these heterogeneous tumors can be observed both inside and outside the treated area, and metastases can occur at more distal locations. Therefore, treatment of head and neck cancers requires effective systemic treatment in addition to the standard surgical and radiation treatments. The

M.A.N. Sendur, MD
Department of Medical Oncology, Yıldırım Beyazıt University,
Faculty of Medicine, Ankara, Turkey

S. Aksoy, MD (✉)
Department of Medical Oncology, Hacettepe University, Cancer Institute,
Sihhiye, Ankara 06100, Turkey
e-mail: saksoy07@yahoo.com

© Springer International Publishing Switzerland 2015
M. Beyzadeoglu et al. (eds.), *Radiation Therapy for Head and Neck Cancers:
A Case-Based Review*, DOI 10.1007/978-3-319-10413-3_2

main aim of multimodal treatment approach is to improve locoregional control and improve survival as well as to achieve preservation of the organ. The use of antineoplastic chemotherapy for patients with potentially curable, advanced, and locoregional disease is generally distinguished from the treatment of recurrent or metastatic stages of disease. Neoadjuvant treatment strategies for tumor reduction before surgery have yet to gain acceptance in locoregionally advanced head and neck squamous cell cancers. But the optimal sequencing of chemotherapy, radiotherapy, and surgery has still remained a subject of controversy for several decades. Concomitant chemoradiotherapy has been shown to improve survival and is considered a standard treatment for locoregionally advanced head and neck squamous cell cancers. Induction chemotherapy protocols before radiotherapy have been used in patients with high risk of distant metastases or for extensive laryngeal cancers, prior to definitive treatment. Despite the improvement of therapeutic management of head and neck cancers, mortality rates of this patients remains high. Thus, molecular targeted therapies have been developed to help increase specificity and reduce toxicity. Targeting epidermal growth factor receptor (EGFR) with specific antibodies has shown clinical activity in palliative and curative settings of head and neck cancers. But the benefit of EGFR antibodies was small; thus, other EGFR inhibitors and novel biologicals of molecular pathways of head and neck cancer are currently being evaluated either as single agents or in combination with other treatment modalities in patients with advanced or metastatic head and neck cancers.

1   Introduction

Head and neck cancers refer to heterogeneous group of tumors extending from the lips to the lower esophagus. Squamous cell cancer is the most common histologic variant, accounting approximately 90–95 % of head and neck cancers. The incidence of head and neck cancer still continues to increase worldwide with approximately half million cases per year [1]. In the United States, it is estimated about 55,070 new head and neck cancers will occur in 2014 which account for up to 3 % of cancer cases [2]. In 2014, it is estimated that 12,000 deaths will occur from head and neck cancer in the United States. In Europe, it is estimated about 139,000 new cases of head and neck cancer per year [3]. In Europe, the 1-year survival rate was 72 %, whereas 5-year survival rate was only 42 % for head and neck cancers in adults [3].

Multidisciplinary approach should be used in all head and neck cancers. The choice of treatment of head and neck cancers depends on the site of the primary tumor, extension of the disease, or the aim of organ preservation. The use of antineoplastic chemotherapy for patients with potentially curable, advanced, and locoregional disease is generally distinguished from the treatment of recurrent or metastatic stages of disease. Approximately 30–40 % of the American Joint Committee on Cancer (AJCC) early-stage I/II head and neck cancers are usually treated with single modality such as radiotherapy or surgery with similar outcomes. Despite single-modality treatment is recommended for early-stage patients, multimodality treatment approaches are recommended for approximately 60 % of AJCC stages III and IV patients [4]. The aim of using chemotherapy with multimodality treatment is to increase cure rates in patients with inoperable or advanced head and neck cancer patients. Neoadjuvant treatment strategies for tumor reduction before surgery have yet to gain acceptance in locoregionally advanced head and neck squamous cell cancers. But the optimal sequencing of chemotherapy, radiotherapy, and surgery has still remained a subject of controversy for several decades [4, 5].

Many chemotherapeutic agents have shown activity as single agents in the metastatic setting squamous cell carcinoma of the head and neck (SCCHN) cancer, but platinum-based chemotherapy consisting of either cisplatin or carboplatin is the recommended first-line treatment for inoperable recurrent or metastatic SCCHN [4, 6]. Targeting epidermal growth factor receptor (EGFR) with specific antibodies have shown clinical activity in palliative and curative settings of head and neck cancers [7–9]. But the benefit of EGFR antibodies was small; thus, other EGFR inhibitors and novel biologicals of molecular pathways of head and neck cancer are currently being evaluated either as single agents or in combination with other treatment modalities in patients with advanced or metastatic head and neck cancers [5].

2   Concurrent Chemotherapy and Radiotherapy

The treatment alternatives continue to improve in patients with locally advanced HNSCC. In early 1990s, 157 previously untreated patients with advanced squamous HNSCC randomly treated with alternating chemotherapy and radiotherapy or radiotherapy alone [10]. In this study, complete response rate was 43 and 22 % ($P=0.03$) in combined therapy and radiotherapy arms, respectively. The median survival was 16.5 months in the combined therapy group and 11.7 months in the radiotherapy group ($P<0.05$). In the 5-year update of this study, the estimated 5-year overall survival (OS) was 24 and 10 % in combined therapy and radiotherapy arms, respectively ($P=0.01$) [11]. Five-year progression-free survival (PFS) was also significantly better in combination treatment arm (21 % vs. 9 %, $P=0.008$).

In another phase III trial, 295 unresectable HNSCC patients randomly assigned to single daily fractionated radiotherapy or identical radiotherapy with concurrent three cycles bolus cisplatin, given on days 1, 22, and 43 or a split course of single daily fractionated radiotherapy and three cycles of concurrent infusional fluorouracil and bolus cisplatin chemotherapy, 30 Gy given with the first cycle and 30–40 Gy given with the third cycle [12]. The 3-year OS rate was significantly increased with concurrent cisplatin and radiotherapy arms (37 % vs. %23, $P=0.014$) compared to radiotherapy alone arm, whereas no significant survival advantage was observed with split course concurrent arm compared to radiotherapy arm (3-year OS; 27 % vs. 23 %).

A meta-analysis of 63 randomized trials (10,741 patients) between 1965 and 1993 showed absolute 4 % survival benefit at 2 and 5 years with adding chemotherapy in the locoregional treatment of HNSCC [13]. In this meta-analysis, no significant benefit with adjuvant or neoadjuvant treatment was observed. Despite the significant benefit was shown with concomitant chemoradiotherapy, the heterogeneity of the results prohibits clear conclusions. In the updated meta-analysis of 93 randomized trials (17,346 patients) between 1965 and 2000, the hazard ratio of death was 0.88 ($P<0.0001$) with an absolute benefit for chemotherapy of 4.5 % at 5 years [14].

In the chemotherapy database (Meta-Analysis of Chemotherapy in Head, Neck Cancer and Nasopharynx Carcinoma) of 120 randomized trials and about 25,000 patients, concomitant cisplatin-based chemoradiotherapy provided the most significant benefit on locoregional control and survival both in HNSCC and nasopharyngeal carcinomas [15].

Concurrent chemoradiotherapy leads to improve disease control not only in unresectable HNSCC but also in resectable stages III and IV HNSCC compared to radiotherapy alone. In a phase III randomized study, efficacy of radiotherapy versus combination chemotherapy and radiotherapy in resectable stages III and IV HNSCC was compared [16]. In this randomized study, 100 resectable stages III and IV HNSCC patients were randomized to either radiotherapy alone, 68–72 Gy at 1.8–2.0 Gy per day, or to radiotherapy with concurrent chemotherapy, 5-fluorouracil, 1,000 mg/m^2/day and cisplatin 20 mg/m^2/day, both given as continuous intravenous infusions over 4 days beginning on day 1 and day 22 of the radiotherapy. With a median 3-year follow-up, relapse-free survival (RFS) was significantly higher in the combination treatment arm compared to radiotherapy arm alone (67 % vs. 52 %, $P=0.03$). Primary site preservation was achieved in 57 % and 35 % of patients with concurrent chemoradiotherapy and radiotherapy arms, respectively ($P=0.02$). Also hematogenous metastases were significantly lower in concurrent chemoradiotherapy compared to radiotherapy arm alone (10 % vs. 21 %, $P=0.04$). After a median 5-year follow-up, OS was not significant between treatment arms, but 5-year OS was significantly higher in patients with successful primary site preservation in the chemoradiotherapy arm [17]. In summary, the addition of concurrent chemotherapy to definitive radiotherapy in patients with resectable stages III and IV HNSCC improved recurrence-free interval and primary site preservation.

Concurrent chemoradiotherapy also has a beneficial role in the organ-preservation treatment of the larynx and for advanced nasopharyngeal cancer. In a randomized phase III Intergroup R91-11 trial, 547 locally advanced larynx cancer patients were randomly assigned to induction cisplatin plus fluorouracil followed by radiotherapy, radiotherapy with concurrent administration of cisplatin, or radiotherapy alone [18]. Two-year results showed that larynx preservation was achieved in 88 and 75 % in radiotherapy with concurrent cisplatin and induction chemotherapy followed by radiotherapy arms, respectively ($P=0.005$), and 70 % in radiotherapy arm alone ($P<0.0001$). In this study, locoregional control was also significantly better with radiotherapy and concurrent cisplatin (78 % vs. 61 % in induction cisplatin plus fluorouracil followed by radiotherapy and 56 % in radiotherapy alone). In the long-term results with a median 10.8-year follow-up, both chemotherapy arms significantly improved laryngectomy-free survival compared to radiotherapy alone [19]. In summary, in Intergroup R91-11 trial locoregional control and larynx preservation were significantly improved with concomitant chemoradiotherapy compared with the induction arm or radiotherapy alone in advanced larynx cancer.

A randomized phase III trial was designed to compare concurrent chemoradiotherapy with radiotherapy alone in 350 patients with locoregionally advanced nasopharyngeal carcinoma [20]. Two-year PFS was 76 % in the concurrent chemoradiotherapy arm and 69 % in the radiotherapy alone arm ($P=0.10$). The primary end point was not met in this trial, but PFS was significantly prolonged in patients with advanced tumor and node stages. After median 5.5-year follow-up, OS was statistically significant in concurrent chemoradiotherapy arm compared to radiotherapy arm alone (70.3 % vs. 58.6 %, $P=0.49$) [21]. Another phase III randomized study concurrent chemoradiotherapy versus radiotherapy alone for 284 patients with advanced nasopharyngeal carcinoma showed that 5-year OS and PFS were significantly improved with concurrent arm compared to radiotherapy arm alone [22]. A meta-analysis of 1,528 patients with locally advanced nasopharyngeal cancer from 6 randomized trials showed that the addition of chemotherapy to radiotherapy increased both PFS and OS by 34 and 20 % at 4 years after treatment [23]. Another meta-analysis of 1,753 patients with locally advanced nasopharyngeal cancer from eight randomized trials showed 6 % absolute survival benefit at 5 years with the addition of chemotherapy to standard radiotherapy with a median 6-year follow-up [24].

3   Induction Chemotherapy

Concurrent chemoradiotherapy is considered as the standard treatment for locally advanced head and neck cancer of the hypopharynx, oropharynx, and larynx. Multiple phase III trials and meta-analyses showed a significant OS and locoregional control benefit of concurrent chemotherapy with radiotherapy. Although chemoradiotherapy has become the standard treatment approach for patients with locally advanced unresectable HNSCC, induction chemotherapy trials with cisplatin plus fluorouracil or taxane with cisplatin plus fluorouracil regimen followed with radiotherapy or chemoradiotherapy aimed to increase survival, organ preservation, and disease control rate.

A randomized study in patients with a squamous cell carcinoma of the oropharynx for whom curative radiotherapy or surgery was considered feasible and was assigned to neoadjuvant chemotherapy followed by locoregional treatment to the same locoregional treatment without chemotherapy [25]. In chemotherapy arm, three cycles of chemotherapy consisting of cisplatin plus fluorouracil (CF) were delivered every 3 weeks. The median survival was 5.1 years in neoadjuvant treatment group, whereas the median survival was 3.3 years in locoregional treatment arm ($P=0.03$). A meta-analysis of 63 randomized trials showed that the addition of CF regimen to locoregional treatment significantly improved the 5-year survival

(6.5 % absolute survival benefit), whereas no significant benefit of locoregional control was shown with the addition of induction chemotherapy regimens [13].

The results of five randomized controlled trials comparing induction docetaxel plus CF have been published. In phase III, TAX 323 trial, 358 patients with locoregionally advanced or unresectable disease of HNSCC were randomly assigned to docetaxel plus CF (TCF) or CF regimen for four cycles every 3 weeks [26]. Radiotherapy was performed within 4–7 weeks after completing chemotherapy if progression was not developed. The primary end point was PFS. With a median 32.5-month follow-up, the median PFS was 11.0 and 8.2 months in the TCF and CF induction arms, respectively ($P=0.007$). The response rate of induction with TCF was also significantly higher in TCF arm compared to CF arm (68 % vs. 54 %, $P=0.006$). Median OS was 18.8 and 14.5 months with TCF and CF induction arms, respectively ($P=0.02$). A randomized phase III TAX 324 trial, randomly assigned 501 patients with locoregionally advanced or unresectable disease of HNSCC either TCF or CF induction chemotherapy, followed by chemoradiotherapy with weekly carboplatin therapy and radiotherapy for 5 days per week [27]. In TAX 324 trial primary end point was OS. The estimated 3-year survival was 62 and 48 % in TCF and CF induction arms, respectively ($P=0.006$). The median OS was 71 months in TCF arm and 30 months in CF arm ($P=0.006$). In the long-term results of TAX 324 trial, 5-year OS was 52.0 and 42 % in TCF and CF arms, respectively, with a median 72.2-month follow-up [28]. Median OS was 70.6 months in TCF arm and 34.8 months in CF arm ($P=0.014$). Median PFS was also significantly improved with TCF regimen compared to CF regimen (38.1 and 13.2 months, $P=0.011$).

GORTEC trial was conducted as a phase III trial for organ preservation of hypopharynx and larynx [29]. In this trial, patients who had larynx and hypopharynx cancer that required total laryngectomy were randomly assigned to receive three cycles of TCF or CF. Patients who responded to chemotherapy received radiotherapy with or without additional chemotherapy. Patients who did not respond to chemotherapy underwent total laryngectomy followed by radiotherapy with or without additional chemotherapy. The primary end point was 3-year larynx-preservation rate. In TCF arm, 3-year larynx-preservation rate was significantly improved compared to CF arm (70.3 % vs. 57.5 %, $P=0.03$).

An individual patient data meta-analysis of 1,772 patients in five randomized trial demonstrated that TCF regimen was significantly associated with improved survival (absolute 7.4 % benefit at 5 years) compared to CF regimen as induction chemotherapy in locally advanced head and neck cancer [30]. Also, TCF arm was associated with significant improved PFS, locoregional control with reduced distant failure.

In another phase III PARADIGM trial, efficacy of TCF induction chemotherapy followed by concurrent chemoradiotherapy with cisplatin-based concurrent chemoradiotherapy alone in patients with locally advanced head and neck cancer was compared [31]. The primary end point was OS. In TCF arm, 3-year OS was 73 %, whereas 78 % in chemoradiotherapy arm alone ($P=0.77$). A phase III randomized DeCIDE trial was randomly assigned two cycles of TCF induction chemotherapy followed with chemoradiotherapy or chemoradiotherapy alone in patients with N2/

N3 locally advanced HNSCC [32]. The primary end point was OS. In DeCIDE trial, 3-year OS was 75.0 and 73.0 % in induction arm and chemoradiotherapy arms, respectively ($P=0.7$).

Induction chemotherapy with definitive radiotherapy regimens also can be used as an aim for organ preservation of the larynx and hypopharynx. A phase III VALCSG (the Department of Veterans Affairs Laryngeal Cancer Study Group) study randomly assigned 332 patients with previously untreated advanced (stages III or IV) laryngeal squamous carcinoma to receive either three cycles of CF regimen and radiation therapy or surgery and radiation therapy [33]. The estimated 2-year survival was 68 % in both arms with a median of 33-month follow-up ($P=0.98$). Total laryngectomy was avoided in 64 % of patients, and on multivariate analyses, T4 and N2 disease were both significant predictors of local treatment failure. Recurrence pattern was also significantly differed between two treatment arms; local failure significantly higher ($P=0.0005$) and distant metastases significantly lower ($P=0.016$) in the chemotherapy arm compared to the surgery arm. A phase III EORTC (the European Organization for Research and Treatment Cancer) trial aimed to compare a larynx-preservation rate with induction chemotherapy plus definitive radiation therapy in patients previously untreated and operable squamous cell carcinomas of the hypopharynx [34]. In the induction chemotherapy arm, complete response of local disease was reported in 54 % of patients and in 51 % of patients with regional disease. The median survival was 44 and 25 months in induction arm and surgery arms, respectively ($P=0.006$), which was less than superiority margin; thus, two treatment arms were accepted as equal. Larynx preservation was achieved in 42 and 35 % of patients in the 3rd and the 5th year with the induction treatment.

In summary, the individual patient data meta-analysis demonstrated that TCF regimen as induction chemotherapy significantly improved OS, PFS, and and locoregional and distant failure compared to CF for locally advanced HNSCC. But the trials presented in this meta-analysis were heterogeneous studies in terms of study design, used doses of chemotherapy drugs, and use of chemoradiotherapy. The TCF induction followed with concomitant chemoradiotherapy with up-front concomitant chemoradiotherapy trials, DeCIDE and PARADIGM, did not demonstrate a significant difference between treatment arms. The main limitations in PARADIGM trial were the use of different chemoradiotherapy regimens and non-standard split course bifractionated docetaxel plus hydroxyurea-based chemoradiotherapy regimen between two treatment arms. Patients with only N2/N3 disease inclusion was the main limitation of DeCIDE trial. In conclusion, concomitant chemoradiotherapy is still the standard treatment in locoregionally advanced HNSCC. There is no evidence from randomized trials suggesting that TCF followed by chemoradiotherapy is superior to chemoradiotherapy alone. Thus, there is no consensus of optimal sequencing of induction chemotherapy and/or chemoradiotherapy [4]. But, induction chemotherapy with definitive radiotherapy regimens can be used as an aim for organ preservation of the larynx and hypopharynx as in EORTC and VALCSG trials [3]. Phase III trials of induction chemotherapy protocols in locally advanced stages III and IV head cancer are summarized in Table 2.1.

Table 2.1 Phase III trials of induction chemotherapy protocols in locally advanced stages III and IV head cancer

Trial name	N	Study design	Cancer type	Primary end point	Comment
GETTEC [25]	318	Locoregional treatment Locoregional treatment plus CF (cisplatin 100 mg/m² on day 1 followed by 5-FU 1,000 mg/m²/day 1–5 days/3 weeks) for 3 cycles	Oropharynx	OS	Median OS: 5.1 vs. 3.3 years ($P=0.03$)
TAX 323 [26]	358	TCF (docetaxel 75 mg/m², cisplatin 75 mg/m² on day 1 followed by 5-FU 750 mg/m² 1–5 days every 3 weeks) for 4 cycles CF (cisplatin 75 mg/m² on day 1 followed by 5-FU 750 mg/m² 1–5 days every 3 weeks) for 4 cycles[a]	Oral cavity, oropharynx, hypopharynx, larynx	PFS	Median PFS: 11.0 vs. 8.2 months ($P=0.007$)
TAX 324 [27, 28]	501	TCF (docetaxel 75 mg/m², cisplatin 100 mg/m² on day 1 followed by 5-FU 1,000 mg/m² 1–4 days every 3 weeks) for 3 cycles CF (cisplatin 100 mg/m² on day 1 followed by 5-FU 750 mg/m² 1–4 days every 3 weeks) for 3 cycles[b]	Oral cavity, oropharynx, hypopharynx, larynx	OS	Median OS: 70.6 vs. 34.8 months ($P=0.014$)
GORTEC [29]	213	TCF (docetaxel 75 mg/m², cisplatin 75 mg/m² on day 1 followed by 5-FU 750 mg/m² 1–5 days every 3 weeks) for 3 cycles CF (cisplatin 75 mg/m² on day 1 followed by 5-FU 750 mg/m² 1–5 days every 3 weeks) for 3 cycles[c]	Hypopharynx, larynx	3-year larynx-preservation rate	3-year larynx-preservation rate; 70.3 % vs. 57.5 % ($P=0.03$)
PARADIGM [31]	145	TCF (docetaxel 75 mg/m², cisplatin 100 mg/m² on day 1 followed by 5-FU 1,000 mg/m² 1–4 days every 3 weeks) for 3 cycles →Chemoradiotherapy alone[d]	Oral cavity, oropharynx, hypopharynx, larynx	OS	3-year OS: 73 % vs. 78 % ($P=0.77$)

DeCIDE [32]	280	TCF (docetaxel 75 mg/m^2, cisplatin 75 mg/m^2 on day 1 followed by 5-FU 750 mg/m^2 1–5 days every 3 weeks) for 2 cycles Chemoradiotherapy alone[e]	N2/N3 HNSCC	OS	3-year OS: 75 % vs. 73 % (P = 0.70)
VALCSG [33]	332	CF (cisplatin 100 mg/m^2 on day 1 followed by 5-FU 1,000 mg/m^2/day 1–5 days/3 weeks) for 3 cycles Radiotherapy[f]	T2–T4 larynx	OS	2-year OS: 68 % in both arms (P = 0.98)
EORTC 24891 [34]	202	CF (cisplatin 100 mg/m^2 on day 1 followed by 5-FU 1,000 mg/m^2/day 1–5 days/3 weeks) for 2–3 cycles Surgery plus radiotherapy[g]	Hypopharynx	Non-inferiority	Median OS: 44 months vs. 25 months (P = 0.006) Non-inferior

[a]Radiotherapy was performed within 4–7 weeks after completing chemotherapy if progression was not developed

[b]All patients were assigned to receive chemoradiotherapy beginning 3–8 weeks after the start of the third cycle of induction chemotherapy. Weekly carboplatin at an area under the curve of 1.5 was given as an intravenous infusion during a 1-h period for a maximum of seven weekly doses during the course of radiotherapy

[c]Patients who responded to chemotherapy received radiotherapy with or without additional chemotherapy

[d]The chemoradiotherapy group consisted of two doses of cisplatin at 100 mg/m^2 given on days 1 and 22 of radiation therapy. TCF arm followed by chemoradiotherapy with docetaxel or carboplatin. Radiotherapy was given as accelerated concomitant boost over 6 weeks or radiotherapy was given once daily over 7 weeks

[e]Chemoradiotherapy alone: [5 days of docetaxel (25 mg/m^2), fluorouracil (600 mg/m^2), hydroxyurea (500 mg BID), and RT (150 cGy BID) followed by a 9-day break] or to two cycles of induction chemotherapy followed by the same CRT

[f]The clinical tumor response was assessed after two cycles of chemotherapy and patients with a response received a third cycle followed by definitive radiation therapy (6,600–7,600 cGy). Patients in whom there was no tumor response or who had locally recurrent cancers after chemotherapy and radiation therapy underwent salvage laryngectomy

[g]An endoscopic evaluation was performed after each cycle of chemotherapy. After two cycles, only partial and complete responders received a third cycle. Patients with a complete response after two or three cycles of chemotherapy were treated thereafter by irradiation (70 Gy); nonresponding patients underwent conventional surgery with postoperative radiation (50–70 Gy)

4   Adjuvant Chemotherapy/Radiotherapy

Many factors can influence survival and locoregional control after primary treatment of head and neck cancers. In two randomized trials, the role of adjuvant chemoradiation was clarified. In randomized EORTC 22931 trial, 334 patients with resected locally advanced head and neck cancer were randomly assigned to radiotherapy alone or with concomitant cisplatin (100 mg/m², on days 1, 22, and 43 of radiotherapy) [35]. High-risk disease was defined as T3 or T4 primary with any nodal stage (except T3N0 laryngeal cancer), positive surgical margins, positive extracapsular extension, positive perineural invasion, or vascular invasion. In EORTC trial, 5-year PFS, OS, and locoregional control were significantly improved in postoperative concurrent chemoradiotherapy arm compared to postoperative radiotherapy alone arm (47 % vs. 36 %; $P=0.04$, 53 % 40 %; $P=0.02$ and 82 % vs. 69; $P=0.007$, respectively) with a median 60-month follow-up.

In RTOG (the Radiation Therapy Oncology Group) 9501 trial, 459 patients with resected high-risk HNSCC randomly assigned to radiotherapy alone or the same doses of RT with concomitant cisplatin (100 mg/m², on days 1, 22, and 43 of radiotherapy) as EORTC trial [36]. In RTOG 9501 trial, high-risk factors were defined as positive surgical margins, positive two or more lymph nodes, or extracapsular nodal extension. In concurrent chemoradiotherapy arm, 2-year locoregional control and DFS were significantly improved compared to radiotherapy arm alone but OS did not differ significantly between treatment groups with a median of 45.9-month follow-up. In the updated results of RTOG 9501 trial at 10 years, locoregional control and DFS were significantly improved only in patients with extracapsular nodal spread or positive margins [37].

In the combined analysis of EORTC 22931 and RTOG 9501 trials for defining risk levels in operated locally advanced HNSCC, extracapsular nodal extension and/or positive surgical margins were found the only risk factors associated with the benefit of concomitant adjuvant chemotherapy and radiotherapy [38]. Thus, the presence of extracapsular nodal extension and/or positive surgical margins is considered a definitive indication of adjuvant treatment according to the current guidelines [3, 4].

5   Systemic Chemotherapy for Metastatic Head and Neck Cancer

The median OS was generally less than 1 year for incurable recurrent or metastatic HNSCC despite intensive chemotherapy and targeted agents [6]. Cisplatin, carboplatin, docetaxel, paclitaxel, methotrexate, fluorouracil, capecitabine, and pemetrexed are commonly used single agents for palliative treatment of incurable recurrent or metastatic HNSCC patients [4]. Despite platinum doublets studies in phase III trials significantly improved response rate, no significant effect on OS was observed [39, 40]. Also no specific platin-based regimen superior to another platin-based regimen despite adding different schedules of taxanes [6, 41]. In symptomatic patients, to increase response rate, platinum-based, multi-agent combination regimens can be given, and single-agent chemotherapy regimens can be given to asymptomatic patients with low tumor burden.

6   EGFR Inhibitors for HNSCC

Overexpression of EGFR was observed approximately in 90 % of HNSCC patients and is associated with poor prognosis [5, 42]. EGFR gene amplification was also associated with poor survival and locoregional recurrence in head and neck cancer. Cetuximab is a chimeric IgG1 monoclonal antibody that specifically binds to EGFR. Cetuximab inhibits DNA double-strand break repair that demonstrates synergistic activity with chemotherapy and radiotherapy [43].

In a randomized phase III trial, 424 patients with locoregionally advanced head and neck cancer were randomly assigned to treatment with high-dose radiotherapy alone or high-dose radiotherapy plus weekly cetuximab [8]. Cetuximab was initiated as loading dose 400 mg/m^2 1 week before radiotherapy followed by a weekly dose of 250 mg/m^2 during radiotherapy. The primary end point of this study was the duration of control of locoregional disease. Locoregional control was significantly improved in patients treated with cetuximab plus radiotherapy compared to radiotherapy alone arm (24.4 months vs. 14.9 months, $P=0.005$). The median OS also significantly improved in cetuximab plus radiotherapy compared to radiotherapy alone arm with a median 54-month follow-up (49.0 months vs. 29.3 months, $P=0.03$). In the subgroup analysis, the beneficial effect was prominent especially oropharyngeal cancers. In the long-term evaluation of this trial, 5-year OS was 45.6 and 36.4 % in cetuximab plus radiotherapy and radiotherapy alone arms, respectively ($P=0.018$) [9]. Additionally, OS benefit was limited to only patients who developed an acneiform rash of at least grade 2 severity.

In phase III EXTREME trial, 442 patients with incurable or metastatic HNSCC randomly assigned to receive platinum-based therapy alone or in combination with cetuximab as a first-line palliative regimen [7]. In cetuximab plus chemotherapy arm, cetuximab monotherapy was given until disease progression or unacceptable toxicity if at least stable disease was achieved after a maximum of six cycles of chemotherapy. The primary end point was OS. EXTREME trial demonstrated a significant OS benefit with the addition of cetuximab to platinum-based therapy; median OS improved from 7.4 to 10.1 months ($P=0.04$).

The OS benefit of cetuximab was shown either as curative treatment or palliative treatment. Cetuximab is the only targeted therapy to be routinely used in clinical practice in the treatment of recurrent or metastatic HNSCC. Other EGFR agents and various biologic agents are under study. Several phase III trials of both cetuximab and novel targeting agents are still ongoing.

Conclusion

Multidisciplinary approach should be used in all head and neck cancers. The choice of treatment of head and neck cancers depends on the site of the primary tumor, the extension of the disease, or the aim of organ preservation. The use of antineoplastic chemotherapy for patients with potentially curable, advanced, and locoregional disease is generally distinguished from the treatment of recurrent or metastatic stages of disease. The aim of using chemotherapy with multimodality treatment is to increase cure rates in patients with inoperable or advanced head and neck cancer patients. Molecular targeted therapies have been developed to help increase specificity and reduce toxicity. Anti-EGFR antibodies have shown clinical activity in palliative and curative settings of head and neck cancers, and other EGFR inhibitors and novel biologicals of molecular pathways of head and neck cancer are currently being evaluated either as single agents or in combination with other treatment modalities in patients with advanced or metastatic head and neck cancers.

References

1. Parkin DM, Bray F, Ferlay J, Pisani P (2005) Global cancer statistics, 2002. CA Cancer J Clin 55(2):74–108
2. Siegel R, Ma J, Zou Z, Jemal A (2014) Cancer statistics, 2014. CA Cancer J Clin 64(1):9–29. doi:10.3322/caac.21208
3. Gregoire V, Lefebvre JL, Licitra L, Felip E, Group E-E-EGW (2010) Squamous cell carcinoma of the head and neck: EHNS-ESMO-ESTRO Clinical Practice Guidelines for diagnosis, treatment and follow-up. Ann Oncol 21(Suppl 5):v184–v186. doi:10.1093/annonc/mdq185
4. Pfister DG, Ang KK, Brizel DM, Burtness BA, Busse PM, Caudell JJ, Cmelak AJ, Colevas AD, Dunphy F, Eisele DW, Gilbert J, Gillison ML, Haddad RI, Haughey BH, Hicks WL Jr, Hitchcock YJ, Kies MS, Lydiatt WM, Maghami E, Martins R, McCaffrey T, Mittal BB, Pinto HA, Ridge JA, Samant S, Schuller DE, Shah JP, Spencer S, Weber RS, Wolf GT, Worden F, Yom SS, McMillian NR, Hughes M, National Comprehensive Cancer N (2013) Head and neck cancers, version 2.2013. Featured updates to the NCCN guidelines. J Natl Compr Canc Netw 11(8):917–923
5. Schmitz S, Ang KK, Vermorken J, Haddad R, Suarez C, Wolf GT, Hamoir M, Machiels JP (2014) Targeted therapies for squamous cell carcinoma of the head and neck: current knowledge and future directions. Cancer Treat Rev 40(3):390–404. doi:10.1016/j.ctrv.2013.09.007
6. Price KA, Cohen EE (2012) Current treatment options for metastatic head and neck cancer. Curr Treat Options Oncol 13(1):35–46. doi:10.1007/s11864-011-0176-y
7. Vermorken JB, Mesia R, Rivera F, Remenar E, Kawecki A, Rottey S, Erfan J, Zabolotnyy D, Kienzer HR, Cupissol D, Peyrade F, Benasso M, Vynnychenko I, De Raucourt D, Bokemeyer C, Schueler A, Amellal N, Hitt R (2008) Platinum-based chemotherapy plus cetuximab in head and neck cancer. N Engl J Med 359(11):1116–1127. doi:10.1056/NEJMoa0802656
8. Bonner JA, Harari PM, Giralt J, Azarnia N, Shin DM, Cohen RB, Jones CU, Sur R, Raben D, Jassem J, Ove R, Kies MS, Baselga J, Youssoufian H, Amellal N, Rowinsky EK, Ang KK (2006) Radiotherapy plus cetuximab for squamous-cell carcinoma of the head and neck. N Engl J Med 354(6):567–578. doi:10.1056/NEJMoa053422
9. Bonner JA, Harari PM, Giralt J, Cohen RB, Jones CU, Sur RK, Raben D, Baselga J, Spencer SA, Zhu J, Youssoufian H, Rowinsky EK, Ang KK (2010) Radiotherapy plus cetuximab for locoregionally advanced head and neck cancer: 5-year survival data from a phase 3 randomised trial, and relation between cetuximab-induced rash and survival. Lancet Oncol 11(1):21–28. doi:10.1016/S1470-2045(09)70311-0
10. Merlano M, Vitale V, Rosso R, Benasso M, Corvo R, Cavallari M, Sanguineti G, Bacigalupo A, Badellino F, Margarino G et al (1992) Treatment of advanced squamous-cell carcinoma of the head and neck with alternating chemotherapy and radiotherapy. N Engl J Med 327(16):1115–1121. doi:10.1056/NEJM199210153271602

11. Merlano M, Benasso M, Corvo R, Rosso R, Vitale V, Blengio F, Numico G, Margarino G, Bonelli L, Santi L (1996) Five-year update of a randomized trial of alternating radiotherapy and chemotherapy compared with radiotherapy alone in treatment of unresectable squamous cell carcinoma of the head and neck. J Natl Cancer Inst 88(9):583–589
12. Adelstein DJ, Li Y, Adams GL, Wagner H Jr, Kish JA, Ensley JF, Schuller DE, Forastiere AA (2003) An intergroup phase III comparison of standard radiation therapy and two schedules of concurrent chemoradiotherapy in patients with unresectable squamous cell head and neck cancer. J Clin Oncol 21(1):92–98
13. Pignon JP, Bourhis J, Domenge C, Designe L (2000) Chemotherapy added to locoregional treatment for head and neck squamous-cell carcinoma: three meta-analyses of updated individual data. MACH-NC Collaborative Group. Meta-Analysis of Chemotherapy on Head and Neck Cancer. Lancet 355(9208):949–955
14. Pignon JP, le Maitre A, Maillard E, Bourhis J, Group M-NC (2009) Meta-analysis of chemotherapy in head and neck cancer (MACH-NC): an update on 93 randomised trials and 17,346 patients. Radiother Oncol 92(1):4–14. doi:10.1016/j.radonc.2009.04.014
15. Bourhis J, Le Maitre A, Baujat B, Audry H, Pignon JP, Meta-Analysis of Chemotherapy in Head NCCG, Meta-Analysis of Radiotherapy in Carcinoma of Head NCG, Meta-Analysis of Chemotherapy in Nasopharynx Carcinoma Collaborative G (2007) Individual patients' data meta-analyses in head and neck cancer. Curr Opin Oncol 19(3):188–194. doi:10.1097/CCO.0b013e3280f01010
16. Adelstein DJ, Saxton JP, Lavertu P, Tuason L, Wood BG, Wanamaker JR, Eliachar I, Strome M, Van Kirk MA (1997) A phase III randomized trial comparing concurrent chemotherapy and radiotherapy with radiotherapy alone in resectable stage III and IV squamous cell head and neck cancer: preliminary results. Head Neck 19(7):567–575
17. Adelstein DJ, Lavertu P, Saxton JP, Secic M, Wood BG, Wanamaker JR, Eliachar I, Strome M, Larto MA (2000) Mature results of a phase III randomized trial comparing concurrent chemoradiotherapy with radiation therapy alone in patients with stage III and IV squamous cell carcinoma of the head and neck. Cancer 88(4):876–883
18. Forastiere AA, Goepfert H, Maor M, Pajak TF, Weber R, Morrison W, Glisson B, Trotti A, Ridge JA, Chao C, Peters G, Lee DJ, Leaf A, Ensley J, Cooper J (2003) Concurrent chemotherapy and radiotherapy for organ preservation in advanced laryngeal cancer. N Engl J Med 349(22):2091–2098. doi:10.1056/NEJMoa031317
19. Forastiere AA, Zhang Q, Weber RS, Maor MH, Goepfert H, Pajak TF, Morrison W, Glisson B, Trotti A, Ridge JA, Thorstad W, Wagner H, Ensley JF, Cooper JS (2013) Long-term results of RTOG 91-11: a comparison of three nonsurgical treatment strategies to preserve the larynx in patients with locally advanced larynx cancer. J Clin Oncol 31(7):845–852. doi:10.1200/JCO.2012.43.6097
20. Chan AT, Teo PM, Ngan RK, Leung TW, Lau WH, Zee B, Leung SF, Cheung FY, Yeo W, Yiu HH, Yu KH, Chiu KW, Chan DT, Mok T, Yuen KT, Mo F, Lai M, Kwan WH, Choi P, Johnson PJ (2002) Concurrent chemotherapy-radiotherapy compared with radiotherapy alone in locoregionally advanced nasopharyngeal carcinoma: progression-free survival analysis of a phase III randomized trial. J Clin Oncol 20(8):2038–2044
21. Chan AT, Leung SF, Ngan RK, Teo PM, Lau WH, Kwan WH, Hui EP, Yiu HY, Yeo W, Cheung FY, Yu KH, Chiu KW, Chan DT, Mok TS, Yau S, Yuen KT, Mo FK, Lai MM, Ma BB, Kam MK, Leung TW, Johnson PJ, Choi PH, Zee BC (2005) Overall survival after concurrent cisplatin-radiotherapy compared with radiotherapy alone in locoregionally advanced nasopharyngeal carcinoma. J Natl Cancer Inst 97(7):536–539. doi:10.1093/jnci/dji084
22. Lin JC, Jan JS, Hsu CY, Liang WM, Jiang RS, Wang WY (2003) Phase III study of concurrent chemoradiotherapy versus radiotherapy alone for advanced nasopharyngeal carcinoma: positive effect on overall and progression-free survival. J Clin Oncol 21(4):631–637
23. Huncharek M, Kupelnick B (2002) Combined chemoradiation versus radiation therapy alone in locally advanced nasopharyngeal carcinoma: results of a meta-analysis of 1,528 patients from six randomized trials. Am J Clin Oncol 25(3):219–223

24. Baujat B, Audry H, Bourhis J, Chan AT, Onat H, Chua DT, Kwong DL, Al-Sarraf M, Chi KH, Hareyama M, Leung SF, Thephamongkhol K, Pignon JP, Group M-NC (2006) Chemotherapy in locally advanced nasopharyngeal carcinoma: an individual patient data meta-analysis of eight randomized trials and 1753 patients. Int J Radiat Oncol Biol Phys 64(1):47–56. doi:10.1016/j.ijrobp.2005.06.037
25. Domenge C, Hill C, Lefebvre JL, De Raucourt D, Rhein B, Wibault P, Marandas P, Coche-Dequeant B, Stromboni-Luboinski M, Sancho-Garnier H, Luboinski B, French Groupe d'Etude des Tumeurs de la Tete et du C (2000) Randomized trial of neoadjuvant chemotherapy in oropharyngeal carcinoma. French Groupe d'Etude des Tumeurs de la Tete et du Cou (GETTEC). Br J Cancer 83(12):1594–1598. doi:10.1054/bjoc.2000.1512
26. Vermorken JB, Remenar E, van Herpen C, Gorlia T, Mesia R, Degardin M, Stewart JS, Jelic S, Betka J, Preiss JH, van den Weyngaert D, Awada A, Cupissol D, Kienzer HR, Rey A, Desaunois I, Bernier J, Lefebvre JL, Group ETS (2007) Cisplatin, fluorouracil, and docetaxel in unresectable head and neck cancer. N Engl J Med 357(17):1695–1704. doi:10.1056/NEJMoa071028
27. Posner MR, Hershock DM, Blajman CR, Mickiewicz E, Winquist E, Gorbounova V, Tjulandin S, Shin DM, Cullen K, Ervin TJ, Murphy BA, Raez LE, Cohen RB, Spaulding M, Tishler RB, Roth B, Viroglio Rdel C, Venkatesan V, Romanov I, Agarwala S, Harter KW, Dugan M, Cmelak A, Markoe AM, Read PW, Steinbrenner L, Colevas AD, Norris CM Jr, Haddad RI, Group TAXS (2007) Cisplatin and fluorouracil alone or with docetaxel in head and neck cancer. N Engl J Med 357(17):1705–1715. doi:10.1056/NEJMoa070956
28. Lorch JH, Goloubeva O, Haddad RI, Cullen K, Sarlis N, Tishler R, Tan M, Fasciano J, Sammartino DE, Posner MR, Group TAXS (2011) Induction chemotherapy with cisplatin and fluorouracil alone or in combination with docetaxel in locally advanced squamous-cell cancer of the head and neck: long-term results of the TAX 324 randomised phase 3 trial. Lancet Oncol 12(2):153–159. doi:10.1016/S1470-2045(10)70279-5
29. Pointreau Y, Garaud P, Chapet S, Sire C, Tuchais C, Tortochaux J, Faivre S, Guerrif S, Alfonsi M, Calais G (2009) Randomized trial of induction chemotherapy with cisplatin and 5-fluorouracil with or without docetaxel for larynx preservation. J Natl Cancer Inst 101(7): 498–506. doi:10.1093/jnci/djp007
30. Blanchard P, Bourhis J, Lacas B, Posner MR, Vermorken JB, Hernandez JJ, Bourredjem A, Calais G, Paccagnella A, Hitt R, Pignon JP, Meta-Analysis of Chemotherapy in H, Neck Cancer IPCG (2013) Taxane-cisplatin-fluorouracil as induction chemotherapy in locally advanced head and neck cancers: an individual patient data meta-analysis of the meta-analysis of chemotherapy in head and neck cancer group. J Clin Oncol 31(23):2854–2860. doi:10.1200/JCO.2012.47.7802
31. Haddad R, O'Neill A, Rabinowits G, Tishler R, Khuri F, Adkins D, Clark J, Sarlis N, Lorch J, Beitler JJ, Limaye S, Riley S, Posner M (2013) Induction chemotherapy followed by concurrent chemoradiotherapy (sequential chemoradiotherapy) versus concurrent chemoradiotherapy alone in locally advanced head and neck cancer (PARADIGM): a randomised phase 3 trial. Lancet Oncol 14(3):257–264. doi:10.1016/S1470-2045(13)70011-1
32. Cohen EE, Karrison T, Kocherginsky M, Huang CH, Agulnik M, Mittal BB, Yunus F, Samant S, Brockstein B, Raez LE, Mehra R, Kumar P, Ondrey FG, Seiwert TY, Villaflor VM, Haraf DJ, EE V (2012) DeCIDE: a phase III randomized trial of docetaxel (D), cisplatin (P), 5-fluorouracil (F) (TPF) induction chemotherapy (IC) in patients with N2/N3 locally advanced squamous cell carcinoma of the head and neck (SCCHN). J Clin Oncol, 2012 ASCO annual meeting abstracts, vol 30, No 15_suppl (May 20 Suppl), 5500
33. Induction chemotherapy plus radiation compared with surgery plus radiation in patients with advanced laryngeal cancer. The Department of Veterans Affairs Laryngeal Cancer Study Group (1991). N Engl J Med 324(24):1685–1690. doi:10.1056/NEJM199106133242402
34. Lefebvre JL, Chevalier D, Luboinski B, Kirkpatrick A, Collette L, Sahmoud T (1996) Larynx preservation in pyriform sinus cancer: preliminary results of a European Organization for Research and Treatment of Cancer phase III trial. EORTC Head and Neck Cancer Cooperative Group. J Natl Cancer Inst 88(13):890–899

35. Bernier J, Domenge C, Ozsahin M, Matuszewska K, Lefebvre JL, Greiner RH, Giralt J, Maingon P, Rolland F, Bolla M, Cognetti F, Bourhis J, Kirkpatrick A, van Glabbeke M, European Organization for R, Treatment of Cancer T (2004) Postoperative irradiation with or without concomitant chemotherapy for locally advanced head and neck cancer. N Engl J Med 350(19):1945–1952. doi:10.1056/NEJMoa032641
36. Cooper JS, Pajak TF, Forastiere AA, Jacobs J, Campbell BH, Saxman SB, Kish JA, Kim HE, Cmelak AJ, Rotman M, Machtay M, Ensley JF, Chao KS, Schultz CJ, Lee N, Fu KK, Radiation Therapy Oncology Group I (2004) Postoperative concurrent radiotherapy and chemotherapy for high-risk squamous-cell carcinoma of the head and neck. N Engl J Med 350(19):1937–1944. doi:10.1056/NEJMoa032646
37. Cooper JS, Zhang Q, Pajak TF, Forastiere AA, Jacobs J, Saxman SB, Kish JA, Kim HE, Cmelak AJ, Rotman M, Lustig R, Ensley JF, Thorstad W, Schultz CJ, Yom SS, Ang KK (2012) Long-term follow-up of the RTOG 9501/intergroup phase III trial: postoperative concurrent radiation therapy and chemotherapy in high-risk squamous cell carcinoma of the head and neck. Int J Radiat Oncol Biol Phys 84(5):1198–1205. doi:10.1016/j.ijrobp.2012.05.008
38. Bernier J, Cooper JS, Pajak TF, van Glabbeke M, Bourhis J, Forastiere A, Ozsahin EM, Jacobs JR, Jassem J, Ang KK, Lefebvre JL (2005) Defining risk levels in locally advanced head and neck cancers: a comparative analysis of concurrent postoperative radiation plus chemotherapy trials of the EORTC (#22931) and RTOG (# 9501). Head Neck 27(10):843–850. doi:10.1002/hed.20279
39. Jacobs C, Lyman G, Velez-Garcia E, Sridhar KS, Knight W, Hochster H, Goodnough LT, Mortimer JE, Einhorn LH, Schacter L et al (1992) A phase III randomized study comparing cisplatin and fluorouracil as single agents and in combination for advanced squamous cell carcinoma of the head and neck. J Clin Oncol 10(2):257–263
40. Forastiere AA, Metch B, Schuller DE, Ensley JF, Hutchins LF, Triozzi P, Kish JA, McClure S, VonFeldt E, Williamson SK et al (1992) Randomized comparison of cisplatin plus fluorouracil and carboplatin plus fluorouracil versus methotrexate in advanced squamous-cell carcinoma of the head and neck: a Southwest Oncology Group study. J Clin Oncol 10(8):1245–1251
41. Gibson MK, Li Y, Murphy B, Hussain MH, DeConti RC, Ensley J, Forastiere AA, Eastern Cooperative Oncology G (2005) Randomized phase III evaluation of cisplatin plus fluorouracil versus cisplatin plus paclitaxel in advanced head and neck cancer (E1395): an intergroup trial of the Eastern Cooperative Oncology Group. J Clin Oncol 23(15):3562–3567. doi:10.1200/JCO.2005.01.057
42. Kalyankrishna S, Grandis JR (2006) Epidermal growth factor receptor biology in head and neck cancer. J Clin Oncol 24(17):2666–2672. doi:10.1200/JCO.2005.04.8306
43. Milas L, Mason K, Hunter N, Petersen S, Yamakawa M, Ang K, Mendelsohn J, Fan Z (2000) In vivo enhancement of tumor radioresponse by C225 antiepidermal growth factor receptor antibody. Clin Cancer Res 6(2):701–708

Management of the Neck

3

Gokhan Ozyigit, Sezin Yuce Sari, Melis Gultekin, Gozde Yazici, Pervin Hurmuz, and Mustafa Cengiz

Overview

The head and neck region has a rich lymphatic network which is divided into sublevels in order to define the regions for surgical neck dissection and radiotherapy. Head and neck cancers have specific routes for lymphatic spread according to their locations. More than 30 % of head and neck tumors are clinically lymph node positive at the time of diagnosis [1], and more than 30 % of patients who are clinically negative have pathologically involved lymph nodes.

Tumors of certain locations do not require elective nodal treatment, as the risk for lymphatic metastasis is less than 5 % (i.e., small tumors of the lip, T1–T2 tumors of the glottic larynx). For the salivary gland, tonsil, paranasal sinus, and middle ear tumors, small tumors of the buccal mucosa and retromolar trigone, and oral tongue tumors not exceeding midline, ipsilateral neck treatment is adequate, whereas for tumors such as the nasopharynx, supraglottic and infraglottic larynx, hypopharynx, soft palate, and base of tongue, bilateral neck treatment is indicated. In case of ipsilateral positive lymph nodes, contralateral neck is also at risk as the metastatic nodes obstruct the lymphatic trunks.

The risk of lateral retropharyngeal lymph node involvement is related to the primary site and neck stage [2]; the medial retropharyngeal nodes are almost never the site of metastatic disease.

G. Ozyigit, MD (✉) • S.Y. Sari, MD • M. Gultekin, MD • G. Yazici, MD
P. Hurmuz, MD • M. Cengiz, MD
Department of Radiation Oncology, Hacettepe University, Faculty of Medicine,
Sihhiye, Ankara, Turkey
e-mail: gozyigit@hacettepe.edu.tr

© Springer International Publishing Switzerland 2015
M. Beyzadeoglu et al. (eds.), *Radiation Therapy for Head and Neck Cancers:
A Case-Based Review*, DOI 10.1007/978-3-319-10413-3_3

1   Introduction

Once the tumor spreads into a lymph node, it expands the node, and the spherical node becomes rounded. Then, the capsule is invaded, leading to extension to adjacent tissues which is called "extracapsular extension". Extracapsular extension impacts prognosis and survival of patients with head and neck cancers significantly.

Nodal areas in the neck are divided into superficial and deep chains. Retropharyngeal and parapharyngeal nodes constitute the latter. The sternocleidomastoid (SCM) muscle divides the neck into two large triangles. The external jugular vein and the platysma muscle are located superficially, where the internal jugular vein, the carotid artery, and some of the cranial nerves are located deeply to the SCM muscle. There are seven lymph node levels proposed by the American Joint Committee on Cancer (AJCC) for head and neck cancers and are shown by Roman numerals (levels I–VII) [3]. These levels are not recommended to be used for lymphomas. Beside these lymph nodes, supraclavicular, retrostyloid space, retropharyngeal, preauricular, intraparotid, buccal, retroauricular, suboccipital, facial, and mastoid lymph nodes, which are not routinely dissected, may also be involved in head and neck cancers. Retropharyngeal nodes are divided into two as medial and lateral. They extend through the internal carotid arteries medially and finally drain into level II lymph nodes. Certain lymphatics have special names: Virchow's node is used for supraclavicular, Delphian's node is used for the precricoid node, and Rouviere's node is the most superior node in the retropharyngeal region (alongside the jugular foramen, and clinically inaccessible).

Different types of neck dissection are performed for particular sites. In radical neck dissection, levels I–V lymph nodes along with superficial and deep cervical fascia they are located in are removed together with the SCM muscle, omohyoid muscle, submandibular gland, internal and external jugular veins, and cranial nerve (CN) XI (spinal accessory nerve). In modified radical dissection, same levels are removed with both fascia, but internal jugular vein, CN XI, or one or more leaves of SCM muscle are not removed. These two techniques require at least ten nodes to be removed. If other lymphatic groups (such as retropharyngeal, levels VI and VII) or non-lymphatic structures (such as the carotid artery, the skin, or the parotid gland) are also removed, it is called an "extended radical dissection". Selective neck dissection is the technique where one or more levels of lymph nodes are not removed, but at least six nodes should be sent for pathologic evaluation. In supraomohyoid dissection (for small oral cavity tumors) levels I–III, in lateral neck dissection (for larynx, oropharynx, and hypopharynx cancers) levels II–IV, in posterolateral neck dissection levels II–V, and in anterior compartment neck dissection level VI are removed. In superselective neck dissection, only the lymph nodes with the highest potential for spread are removed. Following neck dissection, shunts of lymphatic flow develop towards the opposite neck. Also, a previously irradiated neck may have atypical lymphatic drainage [1].

Risks of clinical and pathological bilateral lymph node metastasis of certain head and neck tumors are shown in Table 3.1 [1, 4–9].

Table 3.1 Risks of clinical and pathological bilateral lymph node metastasis of certain head and tumors

Location	Clinically N+ (%)	Clinically N−, pathologically N+ (%)
Glottic larynx	–	15
Supraglottic larynx	39	26
Piriform sinus	49	59
Pharyngeal wall	50	37
Oral tongue	12	33
Floor of the mouth	27	21
Base of tongue	37	55
Tonsil	16	–

N lymph node

2 Evidence-Based Treatment Approaches

Neck irradiation may be performed in negative necks electively (adjuvant or definitive), and in positive necks either preoperatively or postoperatively [10, 11]. Elective neck radiotherapy (RT) has local control (LC) rates similar to elective neck dissection, and neither has an effect on survival [12, 13]. However, Piedbois et al. showed a survival advantage of elective neck dissection over RT in 233 patients with early-stage oral cavity cancers [14]. The decision between RT and dissection is given according to the treatment method for the primary disease. Indications for an elective neck treatment depend on the stage and the grade of the primary lesion. Radiotherapy (RT) (45–50 Gy) is justified in patients with a 20 % or higher risk of occult lymphatic metastatis. Thus, early lesions of the paranasal sinuses, nasal vestibule and nasal cavity, lip, and glottic larynx do not require elective neck RT [15, 16]. The University of Florida published their results for elective neck RT [17, 18]. They observed neck failure in 5 and 21 % of patients who did and did not receive elective neck RT, respectively.

Neck dissection is indicated following RT in patients with multiple, large, and fixated lymph nodes. If positive lymph nodes regress completely after RT, subsequent neck dissection is not necessary [19–22]. The University of Florida recommends following the patients with CT performed after 4 weeks of the last day of RT, and withholding neck dissection if the risk of residual disease is under 5 % [23].

There are two trials showing the efficacy of neck irradiation with a concomitant boost scheme. Peters et al. treated 100 patients with oropharyngeal cancer who had cervical lymph node metastases [24]. Among 62 patients who had complete response to RT, 7 recurred in the neck. Neck control rate was 86 % at 2 years. Subcutaneous fibrosis rate was not different from a group of patients who received RT and neck dissection. Johnson et al. reported complete response in 72 % of 81 patients with lymph node metastases [25]. Among these, 5 % had recurrence in the neck. 3-year neck control was 94 %, and 86 % for <3-cm and >3-cm lymph nodes, respectively. In Mayo Clinic's study, 5-year neck recurrence-free survivals in patients treated with neck dissection only were 76 % for N1, 60 % for N2, and 69 % overall [26].

If neck dissection is "planned" after RT, doses of 50–70 Gy are delivered according to the size and the mobility of the lymph nodes [27]. If the nodes are fixed and/ or the primary disease is treated with RT, the neck should be treated with RT followed by neck dissection. With a planned dissection following a decreased dose of RT, LC is increased, and complications such as fibrosis and cranial nerve palsy are decreased compared to high-dose RT alone.

If RT is to follow surgery, it is generally performed within 4–6 weeks; however, waiting for 10 weeks at most did not affect LC of the neck negatively [27, 28]. In dissected necks with negative margins, 60–65 Gy are prescribed, whereas higher doses are needed for positive margins or residual disease [28–30].

Chao et al. reported the results of 126 patients with head and neck cancer who were treated with IMRT [31]. They observed that most of neck failures were seen within the high-risk region, which was described as CTV1.

As different doses are prescribed for the primary region and the neck according to the presence of residual disease, lymph node metastatis, or extracapsular extension (ECE), Mohan et al. developed "simultaneous integrated boost" in order to be able to prescribe different doses to different regions without decreasing fraction size [32]. Butler et al. defined "simultaneous modulated accelerated radiation therapy" (SMART) where they prescribed 2.4 Gy to high-risk disease in order to minimize the overall treatment time [33]. In RTOG 00–22 study, patients with early-stage oropharyngeal cancer, who had no chemotherapy, received 66 Gy with daily fraction sizes of 2.2 Gy to primary tumor and metastatic nodes, where subclinical disease received 54–60 Gy with daily fraction sizes of 1.8–2 Gy [34]. They found 2-year local failure (LF) rate of 9 % with grade 2 or higher xerostomia rates of 16 % and other toxicities even less. In the study of Ozyigit et al., 2 and 1.2 Gy daily were prescribed to high-risk and low-risk diseases, respectively [35]. The patients were also receiving chemotherapy. They reported no increase in LF in areas receiving 1.2 Gy daily. However, 2-year disease-free survival (DFS) was lower compared to high-dose areas (78 % vs. 94 %).

The decision for prophylactic neck treatment depends on the probability of occult metastasis. This limit is 20 % or higher for many American centers, whereas in Europe, neck treatment is performed if the risk is 5–10 % or higher [36]. In N0 necks, retropharyngeal (RP) lymph nodes should be included in tumors infiltrating the posterior pharynx wall (e.g., nasopharyngeal, hypopharyngeal, oropharyngeal). In tumors of the subglottic or transglottic larynx, and hypopharynx with extension to the esophagus, level VI nodes should be delineated. In nasopharynx cancer, bilateral levels I–V together with RP lymph nodes should be irradiated. According to Byers, this is also the case for N1 necks without ECE [37].

In the majority of patients with N2b disease, levels I–V should be treated [1]. However, in larynx and oral cavity tumors, one may omit level I and level V lymph nodes, respectively (in case they are not metastatic). This is also the case in postoperative patients. In tumors located in the midline or have bilateral lymph node

Table 3.2 Lymph node positivity rates of specific regions (%)

Region	Level I	Level II	Level III	Level IV	Level V	RP
Nasopharynx	17	94	85	19	61	86
Glottic larynx	6	61	54	30	6	
Supraglottic larynx	6	61	54	30	6	4
Piriform sinus	2	77	57	23	22	9
Pharyngeal wall	11	84	72	40	20	21
Oral tongue	39	73	27	11	0	
Floor of mouth	72	51	29	11	5	
Alveolar ridge and retromolar trigone	38	84	25	10	4	
Base of tongue	19	89	22	10	18	6
Tonsil	8	74	31	14	12	12
Thyroid	0	87	100	100	10	

RP retropharyngeal

drainage, contralateral neck should be treated. In patients with neck dissection who have indication for neck irradiation, levels I–V should be treated with previously described exceptions [1].

Lymph node positivity rates of specific regions are shown in Table 3.2 [1, 2, 4–6, 38, 39].

3   Levels of Drainage for Certain Locations of Tumors

Each head and neck subsite have particular pattern of lymphatic drainage [40]:

- *Level Ia*: This level drains the mid-lower lip, anterior oral tongue, anterior floor of the mouth, anterior alveolar mandibular ridge, and skin of the chin.
- *Level Ib*: These nodes are sentinel to maxillary sinus and oral cavity tumors. They drain submandibular gland, anterior and lower nasal cavity, upper and lower lips, hard and soft palates, nasopharynx, anterior of oral tongue, cheeks, maxillary and mandibular alveolar ridges, medial canthus, and soft tissues of the midface.
- *Level II*: This region contains the sentinel lymph nodes for oropharyngeal, oral cavity, supraglottic laryngeal, hypopharyngeal, and thyroid gland cancers. It also drains lymphatics from the nasopharynx, nasal cavity, glottic and subglottic larynx, salivary glands, paranasal sinuses, face, middle ear, and external auditory canal. Oropharyngeal and nasopharyngeal tumors drain to level IIb lymph nodes.
- *Level III*: These lymph nodes are sentinel for subglottic laryngeal and thyroid gland tumors. They also drain nasopharynx, hypopharynx, oropharynx (tonsils, base of the tongue), supraglottic and glottic larynx, paranasal sinuses, and oral cavity tumors.

- *Level IV*: It drains the larynx, hypopharynx, nasopharynx, and cervical esophagus.
- *Level V*: It drains the nasopharynx, oropharynx (tonsils, base of the tongue), apex of piriform sinus, subglottic larynx, cervical esophagus, thyroid gland, occipital and parietal scalp, postauricular and nuchal regions, and skin of the lateral and posterior neck and shoulder.
- *Level VI*: Prelaryngeal lymph nodes are sentinel for glottic and subglottic laryngeal and thyroid gland tumors. They also drain the hypopharynx, cervical esophagus, and apex of the piriform sinus tumors.
- *Retropharyngeal Nodes*: They are sentinel for ethmoid sinus, nasal cavity, and nasopharynx cancers, but also drain the oropharynx, hypopharynx, supraglottic larynx, maxillary sinus, and soft palate.

4   Radiologic Boundaries for Lymph Node Levels of the Neck

Radiologic boundaries for level I lymph nodes are described in Table 3.3 (Fig. 3.1) [40].

Radiologic boundaries for level II lymph nodes are described in Table 3.4 (Fig. 3.2).

Radiologic boundaries for level III lymph nodes are described in Table 3.5 (Fig. 3.3).

Radiologic boundaries for level IV lymph nodes are described in Table 3.6 (Fig. 3.4).

Radiologic boundaries for level V lymph nodes are described in Table 3.7 (Fig. 3.5).

Radiologic boundaries for level VI lymph nodes are described in Table 3.8 (Fig. 3.6).

Radiologic boundaries for retrostyloid space are described in Table 3.9.

Radiologic boundaries for supraclavicular fossa lymph nodes are described in Table 3.10.

Radiologic boundaries for retropharyngeal lymph nodes are described in Table 3.11 (Fig. 3.7).

Table 3.3 Radiologic boundaries for level I lymph nodes

Levels	Terminology	Borders					
		Cranial	Caudal	Anterior	Posterior	Medial	Lateral
Ia	Submental	Cranial border of mandible	Body of hyoid	Platysma muscle	Body of hyoid		Anterior belly of digastric muscle
Ib	Submandibular	Cranial border of submandibular gland, mylohyoid muscle	Central hyoid bone	Platysma muscle	Posterior border of submandibular gland	Anterior belly of digastric muscle	Mandible, skin, platysma muscle

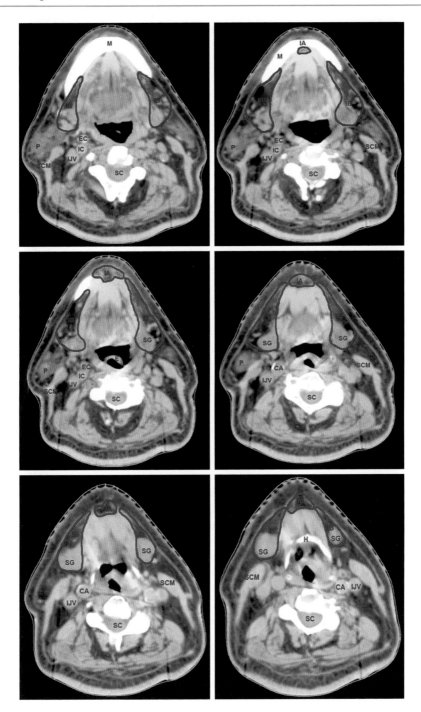

Fig. 3.1 Delineation of level I lymph nodes. Tip: find C1 transverse process to begin level II in case of N(−); otherwise, find jugular foramen (JF) in N(+) neck (see Fig. 3.6 to see JF) (*H* hyoid bone, *IB* level IB, *IA* Level 1A, *SG* submandibular gland, *P* parotid gland, *SC* spinal cord, *IJV* internal jugular vein, *IC* internal carotid artery, *EC* external carotid artery, *CA* common carotid artery, *E* epiglottis, *V* vallecula, *M* mandible, *SCM* sternocleidomastoid muscle)

5   Target Volume Determination and Delineation Guidelines

- *Gross Tumor Volume for Lymph Nodes (GTVn)*: It should include the grossly involved lymph nodes detected by clinical examination, CT, MRI, PET/CT, and intraoperative findings, if operated. In postoperative cases, GTVn is not stated as it is assumed to be grossly resected.
- *Clinical Target Volume for Lymph Nodes (CTVn)*: CTV1 for definitive IMRT is defined as GTV of the primary tumor and GTVn with specific margins. CTV2 is formed by adding high-risk regions for tumor involvement of the primary tumor and metastatic lymph nodes with a 1-cm margin to CTV1. CTV3 includes the uninvolved lymph nodes, and these nodal stations are also called "elective" or "prophylactically treated" nodal regions.
- For postoperative cases, preoperative GTV with 1–2-cm margin including the whole surgical bed and metastatic lymph nodes with ECE is defined as CTV1. CTV2 includes the uninvolved lymph nodes, which are the elective nodal regions in this case. In regions adjacent to parotid glands, deep lobes of the glands are not delineated as critical organs to prevent a decrease in LC in the parapharyngeal space.
- The presence of ECE has a significant importance in terms of LC and survival. Huang et al. reported that patients with ECE required RT in order to improve LC as they have higher risk of recurrence in the neck [41]. In patients with neck dissection and no ECE, CTVn should include wider margins than negative necks, and a 2–3 mm of skin sparing is necessary to decrease skin toxicity [1]. In patients with neck dissection who have ECE, CTVn should have wider margins (including sternocleidomastoid (SCM) and/or paraspinal muscles), and in the regions where there is ECE, the skin is more generously included in CTV. If the muscular fascia is invaded, the entire muscle should be delineated as CTV [40].
- In patients with positive neck, borders of levels differ from the borders in negative necks. If level II lymph nodes are positive, the cranial border starts from the skull base in order to include the jugular fossa. If level IV nodes are positive, the caudal border ends at the clavicular head, to include the supraclavicular region [31].
- In patients with no neck dissection, studies showed that the size of the lymph node is important on estimating the risk of ECE [42–46]. If the lymph node is smaller than 1 cm, the risk of ECE is 17–43 %. However, when it exceeds 3 cm, the risk may rise up to 95 %. As we do not have pathologic evaluation in patients without neck dissection, the size of the nodes should be taken into account, and generous margins should be added for larger ones. A study from MD Anderson Cancer Center reported that margins of 5 and 10 mm are adequate for covering 90 and 100 % of microscopic ECE, respectively [47].
- In 2014, radiation oncologists from the Danish Head and Neck Cancer Group (DAHANCA), the European Organization for Research and Treatment of Cancer (EORTC), the Hong Kong Nasopharyngeal Cancer Study Group (HKNPCSG), the National Cancer Institute of Canada Clinical Trials Group (NCIC CTG), the

Table 3.4 Radiologic boundaries for level II lymph nodes

Levels	Terminology	Borders					
		Cranial	Caudal	Anterior	Posterior	Medial	Lateral
IIa	Upper jugular (jugulodigastric)	Superior border of transverse process of C1 vertebra	inferior border of hyoid bone	Posterior to submandibular gland	Posterior to jugular vein	Medial border of ICA	Medial border of SCM muscle
IIb		Superior border of transverse process of C1 vertebra	Inferior border of hyoid bone	Posterior to jugular vein	Posterior border of SCM muscle	Deep cervical muscles	Medial border of SCM muscle

ICA internal carotid artery, *SCM* sternocleidomastoid

Radiation Therapy Oncology Group (RTOG), and the Trans Tasman Radiation Oncology Group (TROG) published a new recommendation guideline for the delineation of neck node levels with the cooperation of an anatomist and a head and neck surgeon [48].

This recent guidelines divided the neck node levels into ten subsites. There is no significant difference in the description and delineation of levels I, II, and III. However, levels IV, VI, and VII were subdivided into two, whereas level V was subdivided into three subgroups, and levels VIII, IX, and X were recently proposed.

They described level IVa lymph nodes as the previous level IV (e.g., lower jugular lymph nodes) and level IVb as the medial supraclavicular lymph nodes which lie between the anterior border of the scalenus muscle and the apex of the lung. The previously described level V was subdivided into level Va and Vb lymph nodes separated by the caudal edge of the cricoid cartilage. Level Vc was recently proposed for the lateral supraclavicular lymph nodes which lie lateral to the scalenus muscle and lateral border of level IVa. Level VI was also divided into VIa and VIb lymph nodes as anterior jugular, and prelaryngeal, pretracheal, and paratracheal lymph nodes, respectively. The previously defined retropharyngeal and retrostyloid lymph nodes were named as levels VIIa and VIIb, respectively. In level VIIb lymph nodes, lateral retropharyngeal nodes were solely included, excluding the medial nodes. The parotid lymph nodes (e.g., preauricular, intraparotid, and subparotid nodes) were defined as level VIII, whereas the malar and buccofacial nodes were defined as level IX lymph nodes. Level X was subdivided into levels Xa and Xb which contain retro- and subauricular and occipital lymph nodes, respectively.

- *Planning Target Volume (PTV)*: A margin of 3 mm is added in all directions; however, it may be minimized to 1 mm in areas adjacent to critical structures.
- *Guidelines for Clinical Target Volumes of the Neck*
  Guidelines for clinical target volumes of the neck are shown in Table 3.12.
- *Recommendations for Target Volume Dose Prescriptions*
  Recommendations for target volume dose prescriptions are summarized in Table 3.13.

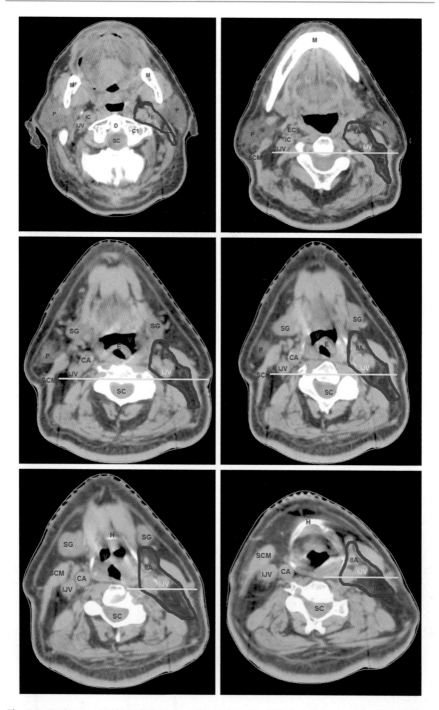

Fig. 3.2 Delineation of level II lymph nodes. Tip: *yellow line* just at the posterior edge of IJV divides level II into A and B. (*SG* submandibular gland, *P* parotid gland, *SC* spinal cord, *IJV* internal jugular vein, *IC* internal carotid artery, *EC* external carotid artery, *CA* common carotid artery, *E* epiglottis, *V* vallecula, *M* mandible, *SCM* sternocleido mastoid muscle, *H* hyoid bone, *D* dens of axis, *C1* C1 cervical vertebrae)

Table 3.5   Radiologic boundaries for level III lymph nodes

Level	Terminology	Borders					
		Cranial	Caudal	Anterior	Posterior	Medial	Lateral
III	Mid-jugular (jugulo-omohyoid)	Inferior to body of hyoid	Inferior to cricoid	Anterior border of SCM muscle	Posterior border of SCM muscle	Medial border of ICA, deep cervical muscles	Lateral border of SCM muscle

ICA internal carotid artery, *SCM* sternocleidomastoid

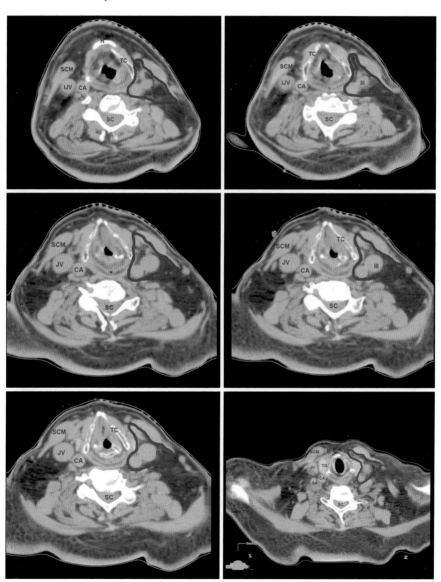

Fig. 3.3   Delineation of level III lymph nodes (*SC* spinal cord, *IJV* internal jugular vein, *CA* common carotid artery, *SCM* sternocleido mastoid muscle, *H* Hyoid bone, *TC* Thyroid cartilage, *Cr* Cricoid cartilage, *TG* Thyroid gland, *SA* Scalenus anterior muscle, *JV* Jugular vein)

Table 3.6 Radiologic boundaries for level IV lymph nodes

Level	Terminology	Borders					
		Cranial	Caudal	Anterior	Posterior	Medial	Lateral
IV	Lower jugular (transverse cervical)	Inferior to cricoid	2 cm superior to sternoclavicular joint	Anteromedial border of SCM muscle	posterior border of SCM muscle	Medial border of ICA, paraspinal muscles	Medial border of SCM muscle

ICA internal carotid artery, *SCM* sternocleidomastoid

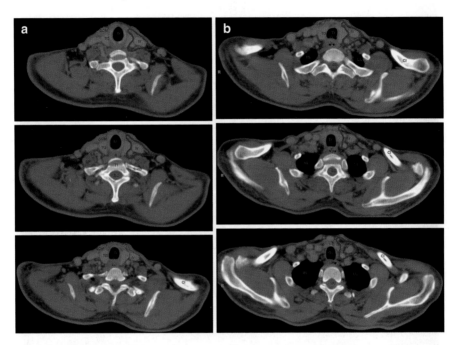

Fig. 3.4 (**a**, **b**) Delineation of level IV lymph nodes (*SC* spinal cord, *SCM* sternocleido mastoid muscle, *H* hyoid bone, *TC* thyroid cartilage, *Cr* cricoid cartilage, *TG* thyroid gland, *SA* scalenus anterior muscle, *SP* scalenus posterior muscle, *Tr* trachea,*T1* T1 vertebrae, *E* esophagus, *Cl* clavicle, *RL* right lung, *LL* left lung)

Table 3.7 Radiologic boundaries for level V lymph nodes

Levels	Terminology	Borders					
		Cranial	Caudal	Anterior	Posterior	Medial	Lateral
Va		Superior to hyoid	Inferior border of cricoid	Posterior border of SCM muscle	Anterolateral border of trapezius muscle	Deep paraspinal muscles	Skin, platysma
Vb	Spinal accessory chain (posterior triangle)	Inferior border of cricoid	Transverse cervical arteries	Posterior border of SCM muscle	Anterolateral border of trapezius muscle	Deep paraspinal muscles	Skin, platysma

SCM sternocleidomastoid

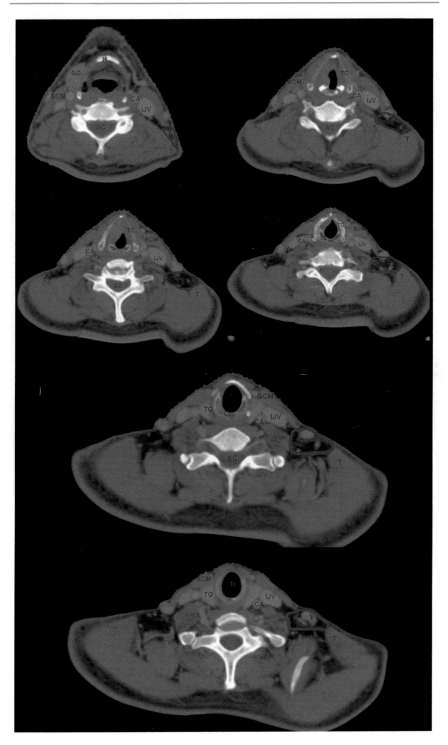

Fig. 3.5 Delineation of level V lymph nodes (*SG* submandibular gland, *SC* spinal cord, *IJV* internal jugular vein, *CA* common carotid artery, *SCM* sternocleido mastoid muscle, *PS* pyriform sinus, *T* trapezius muscle, *tc* transverse cervical vessels, *TG* thyroid gland, *TC* thyroid cartilage, *Cr* cricoid cartilage)

Table 3.8 Radiologic boundaries for level VI lymph nodes

Level	Terminology	Borders					
		Cranial	Caudal	Anterior	Posterior	Medial	Lateral
VI	Anterior compartment (prelaryngeal, pretracheal, precricoid, and tracheoesophageal)	Superior to thyroid/caudal edge of cricoid cartilage (for paratracheal nodes)	Manubrium of sterni	Skin/ cricoid cartilage (for pretracheal nodes)	Esophagus/ trachea	Trachea	Medial border of SCM muscle, thyroid gland

SCM sternocleidomastoid muscle

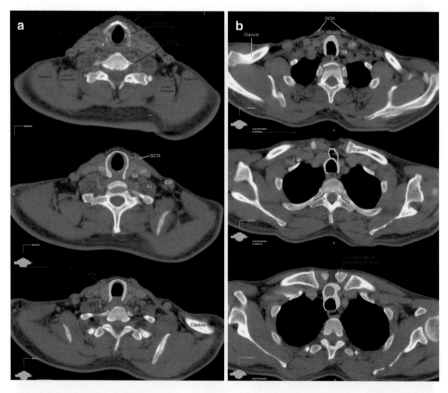

Fig. 3.6 Delineation of level VI lymph nodes (Level VIa *red*, Level IVb *aqua*). (*EJV* external jugular vein, *IJV* internal jugular vein, *CA* common carotid artery, *SCM* sternocleido mastoid muscle, *Sc* scalenius muscle, *E* esophagus, *TG* thyroid gland, *LCo* longus colli muscle, *LCa* longus capitis muscle)

Table 3.9 Radiologic boundaries for retrostyloid space

Level	Terminology	Borders					
		Cranial	Caudal	Anterior	Posterior	Medial	Lateral
RSS	Retrostyloid space	Base of skull (jugular foramen)	Upper limit level II	Parapharyngeal space	Vertebra, base of skull	Retropharygeal nodes	Parotid space

Table 3.10 Radiologic boundaries for supraclavicular fossa lymph nodes

Level	Terminology	Borders					
		Cranial	Caudal	Anterior	Posterior	Medial	Lateral
SCF	Supraclavicular	Lower border of IV/Vb	Sternoclavicular joint	SCM muscle, skin, clavicle	Anterior border of posterior scalenus muscle	Trachea/thyroid	Lateral border of posterior scalenus muscle

Table 3.11 Radiologic boundaries for retropharyngeal lymph nodes

Level	Terminology	Borders					
		Cranial	Caudal	Anterior	Posterior	Medial	Lateral
RP	Retropharyngeal	Base of skull	Superior border of hyoid bone (level of C3 vertebra)	Fascia, pharynx mucosa	Longus colli/capitus muscles	Midline	Medial border of ICA

ICA internal carotid artery

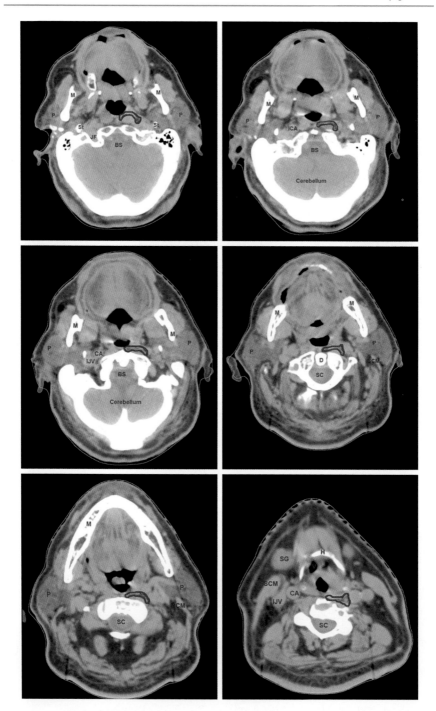

Fig. 3.7 Delineation of retropharyngeal lymph nodes. (*SG* submandibular gland, *P* parotid gland, *SC* spinal cord, *IJV* internal jugular vein, *IC* internal carotid artery, *CA* common carotid artery, *H* hyoid bone, *V* vallecula, *M* mandible, *SCM* sternocleido mastoid muscle, *BS* brain stem, *JF* jugular foramen, *D* Dens of axis, *St* Styloid process)

Table 3.12 Guidelines for clinical target volumes of the neck

Treatment modality	CTV1	CTV2	CTV3
Definitive IMRT	Gross lymph node	Positive lymph node levels	Elective nodal regions
Postoperative IMRT	Positive lymph node levels with ECE	Positive lymph node levels without ECE	Elective nodal regions

IMRT intensity-modulated radiation therapy, *CTV* clinical target volume, *ECE* extracapsular extension

Table 3.13 Recommendations for target volume dose prescriptions

Reference	Concurrent chemotherapy	CTV1	CTV2	CTV3
Butler et al. [33]	–	60/2.4 Gy	–	50/2 Gy
Chao et al. [31]	+	70/2 Gy	59.4/1.8 Gy	56/1.6 Gy
Lee et al. [49]	+	70/2.12 Gy	59.4/1.8 Gy	–
Eisbruch et al. (RTOG H-0022) [34]	–	66/2.2 Gy	60/2 Gy	54/1.8 Gy

CTV clinical target volume

References

1. Chao KS et al (2002) Determination and delineation of nodal target volumes for head-and-neck cancer based on patterns of failure in patients receiving definitive and postoperative IMRT. Int J Radiat Oncol Biol Phys 53(5):1174–1184
2. McLaughlin MP et al (1995) Retropharyngeal adenopathy as a predictor of outcome in squamous cell carcinoma of the head and neck. Head Neck 17(3):190–198
3. Robbins KT et al (2002) Neck dissection classification update: revisions proposed by the American Head and Neck Society and the American Academy of Otolaryngology-Head and Neck Surgery. Arch Otolaryngol Head Neck Surg 128(7):751–758
4. Bataini JP et al (1985) Natural history of neck disease in patients with squamous cell carcinoma of oropharynx and pharyngolarynx. Radiother Oncol 3(3):245–255
5. Byers RM, Wolf PF, Ballantyne AJ (1988) Rationale for elective modified neck dissection. Head Neck Surg 10(3):160–167
6. Lindberg R (1972) Distribution of cervical lymph node metastases from squamous cell carcinoma of the upper respiratory and digestive tracts. Cancer 29(6):1446–1449
7. Northrop M et al (1972) Evolution of neck disease in patients with primary squamous cell carcinoma of the oral tongue, floor of mouth, and palatine arch, and clinically positive neck nodes neither fixed nor bilateral. Cancer 29(1):23–30
8. Woolgar JA (1999) Histological distribution of cervical lymph node metastases from intraoral/oropharyngeal squamous cell carcinomas. Br J Oral Maxillofac Surg 37(3):175–180
9. Buckley JG, MacLennan K (2000) Cervical node metastases in laryngeal and hypopharyngeal cancer: a prospective analysis of prevalence and distribution. Head Neck 22(4):380–385
10. Dubray BM et al (1993) Is reseeding from the primary a plausible cause of node failure? Int J Radiat Oncol Biol Phys 25(1):9–15
11. Mendenhall WM et al (2002) Planned neck dissection after definitive radiotherapy for squamous cell carcinoma of the head and neck. Head Neck 24(11):1012–1018
12. Vandenbrouck C et al (1980) Elective versus therapeutic radical neck dissection in epidermoid carcinoma of the oral cavity: results of a randomized clinical trial. Cancer 46(2):386–390

13. Fakih AR et al (1989) Elective versus therapeutic neck dissection in early carcinoma of the oral tongue. Am J Surg 158(4):309–313
14. Piedbois P et al (1991) Stage I-II squamous cell carcinoma of the oral cavity treated by irid-ium-192: is elective neck dissection indicated? Radiother Oncol 21(2):100–106
15. Mendenhall WM et al (1989) Is elective neck treatment indicated for T2N0 squamous cell carcinoma of the glottic larynx? Radiother Oncol 14(3):199–202
16. Mendenhall WM et al (1988) T1-T2 vocal cord carcinoma: a basis for comparing the results of radiotherapy and surgery. Head Neck Surg 10(6):373–377
17. Mendenhall WM, Million RR (1986) Elective neck irradiation for squamous cell carcinoma of the head and neck: analysis of time-dose factors and causes of failure. Int J Radiat Oncol Biol Phys 12(5):741–746
18. Mendenhall WM, Million RR, Cassisi NJ (1980) Elective neck irradiation in squamous-cell carcinoma of the head and neck. Head Neck Surg 3(1):15–20
19. Bartelink H (1983) Prognostic value of the regression rate of neck node metastases during radiotherapy. Int J Radiat Oncol Biol Phys 9(7):993–996
20. Bartelink H, Breur K, Hart G (1982) Radiotherapy of lymph node metastases in patients with squa-mous cell carcinoma of the head and neck region. Int J Radiat Oncol Biol Phys 8(6):983–989
21. Bataini JP et al (1987) Impact of neck node radioresponsiveness on the regional control prob-ability in patients with oropharynx and pharyngolarynx cancers managed by definitive radio-therapy. Int J Radiat Oncol Biol Phys 13(6):817–824
22. Maciejewski B (1987) Regression rate of metastatic neck lymph nodes after radiation treat-ment as a prognostic factor for local control. Radiother Oncol 8(4):301–308
23. Liauw SL et al (2006) Postradiotherapy neck dissection for lymph node-positive head and neck cancer: the use of computed tomography to manage the neck. J Clin Oncol 24(9):1421–1427
24. Peters LJ et al (1996) Neck surgery in patients with primary oropharyngeal cancer treated by radiotherapy. Head Neck 18(6):552–559
25. Johnson CR et al (1998) Radiotherapeutic management of bulky cervical lymphadenopathy in squamous cell carcinoma of the head and neck: is postradiotherapy neck dissection necessary? Radiat Oncol Investig 6(1):52–57
26. Olsen KD et al (1994) Primary head and neck cancer. Histopathologic predictors of recurrence after neck dissection in patients with lymph node involvement. Arch Otolaryngol Head Neck Surg 120(12):1370–1374
27. Mendenhall WM et al (1988) Squamous cell carcinoma of the head and neck treated with radiation therapy: the impact of neck stage on local control. Int J Radiat Oncol Biol Phys 14(2):249–252
28. Amdur RJ et al (1989) Postoperative irradiation for squamous cell carcinoma of the head and neck: an analysis of treatment results and complications. Int J Radiat Oncol Biol Phys 16(1):25–36
29. Marcus RB Jr, Million RR, Cassissi NJ (1979) Postoperative irradiation for squamous cell carcinomas of the head and neck: analysis of time-dose factors related to control above the clavicles. Int J Radiat Oncol Biol Phys 5(11–12):1943–1949
30. Million RR (1979) Squamous cell carcinoma of the head and neck: combined therapy: surgery and postoperative irradiation. Int J Radiat Oncol Biol Phys 5(11–12):2161–2162
31. Chao KS et al (2003) Patterns of failure in patients receiving definitive and postoperative IMRT for head-and-neck cancer. Int J Radiat Oncol Biol Phys 55(2):312–321
32. Mohan R et al (2000) Radiobiological considerations in the design of fractionation strategies for intensity-modulated radiation therapy of head and neck cancers. Int J Radiat Oncol Biol Phys 46(3):619–630
33. Butler EB et al (1999) Smart (simultaneous modulated accelerated radiation therapy) boost: a new accelerated fractionation schedule for the treatment of head and neck cancer with intensity modulated radiotherapy. Int J Radiat Oncol Biol Phys 45(1):21–32
34. Eisbruch A et al (2010) Multi-institutional trial of accelerated hypofractionated intensity-modulated radiation therapy for early-stage oropharyngeal cancer (RTOG 00–22). Int J Radiat Oncol Biol Phys 76(5):1333–1338

35. Chao KS, Ozyigit G, Thorsdad WL (2003) Toxicity profile of intensity-modulated radiation therapy for head and neck carcinoma and potential role of amifostine. Semin Oncol 30(6 Suppl 18):101–108
36. Weiss MH, Harrison LB, Isaacs RS (1994) Use of decision analysis in planning a management strategy for the stage N0 neck. Arch Otolaryngol Head Neck Surg 120(7):699–702
37. Byers RM (1985) Modified neck dissection. A study of 967 cases from 1970 to 1980. Am J Surg 150(4):414–421
38. Candela FC, Kothari K, Shah JP (1990) Patterns of cervical node metastases from squamous carcinoma of the oropharynx and hypopharynx. Head Neck 12(3):197–203
39. Shah JP, Candela FC, Poddar AK (1990) The patterns of cervical lymph node metastases from squamous carcinoma of the oral cavity. Cancer 66(1):109–113
40. Gregoire V et al (2003) CT-based delineation of lymph node levels and related CTVs in the node-negative neck: DAHANCA, EORTC, GORTEC, NCIC, RTOG consensus guidelines. Radiother Oncol 69(3):227–236
41. Huang DT et al (1992) Postoperative radiotherapy in head and neck carcinoma with extracapsular lymph node extension and/or positive resection margins: a comparative study. Int J Radiat Oncol Biol Phys 23(4):737–742
42. Johnson JT et al (1981) The extracapsular spread of tumors in cervical node metastasis. Arch Otolaryngol 107(12):725–729
43. Snow GB et al (1982) Prognostic factors of neck node metastasis. Clin Otolaryngol Allied Sci 7(3):185–192
44. Snyderman NL et al (1985) Extracapsular spread of carcinoma in cervical lymph nodes. Impact upon survival in patients with carcinoma of the supraglottic larynx. Cancer 56(7):1597–1599
45. Carter RL et al (1987) Radical neck dissections for squamous carcinomas: pathological findings and their clinical implications with particular reference to transcapsular spread. Int J Radiat Oncol Biol Phys 13(6):825–832
46. Hirabayashi H et al (1991) Extracapsular spread of squamous cell carcinoma in neck lymph nodes: prognostic factor of laryngeal cancer. Laryngoscope 101(5):502–506
47. Apisarnthanarax S et al (2006) Determining optimal clinical target volume margins in head-and-neck cancer based on microscopic extracapsular extension of metastatic neck nodes. Int J Radiat Oncol Biol Phys 64(3):678–683
48. Gregoire V et al (2014) Delineation of the neck node levels for head and neck tumors: a 2013 update. DAHANCA, EORTC, HKNPCSG, NCIC CTG, NCRI, RTOG, TROG consensus guidelines. Radiother Oncol 110(1):172–181
49. Lee N et al (2002) Intensity-modulated radiotherapy in the treatment of nasopharyngeal carcinoma: an update of the UCSF experience. Int J Radiat Oncol Biol Phys 53(1):12–22

Nasal Cavity and Paranasal Sinuses

4

Gozde Yazici, Sezin Yuce Sari, Mustafa Cengiz,
Pervin Hurmuz, Melis Gultekin, and Gokhan Ozyigit

Overview

Epidemiology

Tumors of the nasal cavity and paranasal sinuses are relatively uncommon, with an incidence of 0.75/100.000 in the USA [1]. They are usually diagnosed after the age of 40. The nasal cavity consists of four subsites; the nasal vestibule, the lateral walls, the floor, and the septum. Paranasal sinuses are named after their locations as maxillary, ethmoid, sphenoid, and frontal. Tumors originating from the maxillary sinus are the most common among all, having an incidence approximately twice as the nasal cavity tumors. Ethmoid sinus lesions are the second most common tumors, and tumors of other locations are extremely rare. The etiologic factors are comprised of occupational exposure such as wood dust, glues, nickel, chromium, mustard gas, isopropyl alcohol, and radium [2–6]. Thorotrast, an agent historically used in radiographic studies for maxillary sinus imaging, also was associated with maxillary sinus carcinomas. Tobacco and alcohol consumption are shown to increase the risk of nasal cancer.

Pathological and Biological Features

Majority of these tumors are squamous cell carcinomas (SCC). Basal cell carcinoma, adnexal carcinoma, minor salivary gland neoplasms (i.e., adenocarcinoma (the second most common), adenoid cystic carcinoma (the third most common), and mucoepidermoid carcinoma), melanoma, neuroendocrine carcinoma (i.e., small cell carcinoma, esthesioneuroblastoma, and

G. Yazici, MD (✉) • S.Y. Sari, MD • M. Cengiz, MD • P. Hurmuz, MD
M. Gultekin, MD • G. Ozyigit, MD
Department of Radiation Oncology, Faculty of Medicine, Hacettepe University,
Sihhiye, Ankara, Turkey
e-mail: yazicig@hacettepe.edu.tr

© Springer International Publishing Switzerland 2015
M. Beyzadeoglu et al. (eds.), *Radiation Therapy for Head and Neck Cancers:
A Case-Based Review*, DOI 10.1007/978-3-319-10413-3_4

sinonasal undifferentiated carcinoma), lymphoma, sarcoma, and plasmacytoma are less common histopathologic entities.

Definitive Therapy
Radiotherapy is the preferred treatment modality over surgery for tumors of nasal vestibule in order to obtain better cosmesis with equal local control rates. For large tumors with deep invasion, surgery, in combination with neo-adjuvant or adjuvant radiotherapy, is the treatment of choice. For small tumors of ethmoid sinuses and other sites of nasal cavity, results of radiotherapy and surgery are equivalent. Small tumors of maxillary sinuses may be treated with surgery alone. Chemoradiotherapy is an option for patients who refuse surgery.

Adjuvant Therapy
Surgery and adjuvant radiotherapy is the standard treatment for locally advanced maxillary sinus tumors. Postoperative radiotherapy is also indicated for positive surgical margins, lymphatic invasion, or perineural invasion. Chemotherapy has a limited role for the tumors of this region.

1   Case Presentation

A 27-year old male admitted to the hospital with swelling and redness in the left eye. He was also suffering from headache in the frontal region periodically. There was no vision loss or diplopia. He had no significant medical history other than an adenoidectomy 20 years ago.

His physical and endoscopic examination revealed a mass in the left middle meatus. The nasal septum was slightly deviated to the right. Nasal passages were narrowed. The nasopharynx, oropharynx, oral cavity, and larynx were intact. There were no pathologic lymph nodes in his neck.

The MRI detected a giant mass completely obliterating the superior 2/3 portion of the left nasal cavity and eroding the superior nasal conchae (Fig. 4.1). It also invaded the medial wall of the left maxillary sinus and extended through the sinus. The left orbit was invaded via erosion of its medial wall, and medial extraocular muscles were displaced. Lamina papyracea, ethmoid cells, bony structure at the base of frontal lobe, crista galli, cribriform plate, left ethmoid foveae, left half of sphenoid, and frontal sinuses were also invaded with intracranial extension. Multiple conglomerated lymphadenopathies in the left cervical chain and submandibular region were present.

Biopsy from the nasal mucosa revealed undifferentiated carcinoma. Endoscopic resection was performed. The pathology revealed the same histology.

He was diagnosed with T4bN2bM0 maxillary sinus carcinoma.

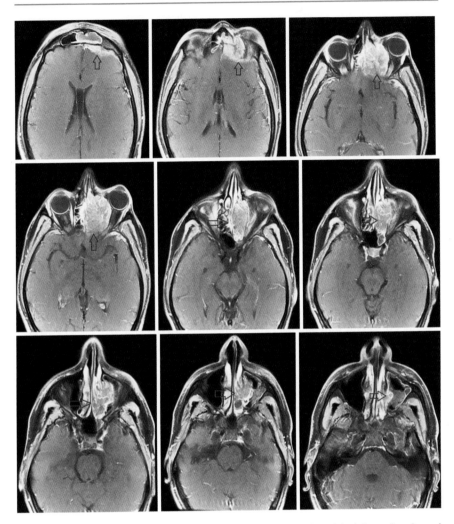

Fig. 4.1 A giant mass completely obliterating the superior 2/3 portion of the left nasal cavity and eroding superior nasal conchae seen on MRI

---

2 Evidence-Based Treatment Approaches

Nasal Vestibule Tumors

Primary radiotherapy (RT) is preferred for small superficial tumors because of cosmetic concerns. However, surgery may also lead to high local control (LC) rates with excellent cosmetic results in selected cases. The size and location of the tumor guide us to choose the appropriate technique of RT. Brachytherapy (BRT) and external beam radiotherapy (EBRT) have similar cure rates reaching to 90 % for tumors up to 2 cm. For tumors larger than 2 cm, higher doses are needed to reach 80 % LC rates [7–11].

Large tumors with deep extensions require surgery in combination with neoadjuvant or adjuvant RT. Mazeron et al. evaluated 1,676 patients with nasal vestibule and skin of the nose cancers who were treated with BRT or EBRT. They reported 93 % overall LC rate. Tumors smaller than 2 cm and located externally (skin of the nose) have better LC rates (96 % for <2 cm vs. 81 % for >4 cm, and 94 % for skin of the nose vs. 75 % for the vestibule). However, LC rate with surgery only was no more than 90 % [12].

Nasal Cavity Tumors

Surgery and RT have similar results for small tumors in terms of cure. Daly et al. reported 91 % 5-year overall survival (OS) rates with either treatment modality [13]. Surgery may be preferred for posterior nasal septum tumors, whereas BRT is the treatment of choice for anterior and inferior septum tumors not larger than 1.5 cm. For lateral wall tumors, EBRT rather than BRT is preferred because of cosmetic concerns. In a study of 45 patients who were treated with solely RT, or RT combined with surgery, 5-year OS rate was 75 % [14]. In this study, Ang et al. reported that lateral wall and floor tumors had inferior prognosis compared to septum tumors (LC rates, 68 % vs. 86 %). For stages II–IVa, surgery should be performed with or without adjuvant RT.

Paranasal Sinus Tumors

Surgery and adjuvant RT are the treatment of choice for ethmoid sinus tumors. If cosmetic or functional result is an issue, RT alone or concurrent chemoradiotherapy (CRT) may be an option [15]. Choussy et al. reported tumor extension, lymph node involvement, and the presence of brain invasion as prognostic factors for ethmoid tumors. They found nearly half of the patients who received adjuvant RT after surgery had recurrences, 75 % of which were local [16]. Blanco et al. reported 5-year LC, DFS, and OS rates as 61, 35, and 29 %, respectively, in 106 patients with paranasal sinus cancers who received RT [17].

Surgery alone is efficient for early-stage maxillary sinus tumors. Adjuvant RT is indicated in patients with locally advanced disease. Combination therapy has better 5-year LC and OS rates than single treatment modalities, both ranging from 44 to 80 %. 5-year LC and OS rates with RT alone were reported as 39 and 40 %, respectively. Parsons et al. reported survival rates of 60, 70, 30, and 40 % for T1, T2, T3, and T4 lesions treated with surgery and RT, respectively [18]. In locally advanced tumors, solely RT results are dismal with 5-year survival rates of 10–15.

Intensity-modulated radiation therapy (IMRT) is accepted as the standard RT modality. A previous study from UCSF observed no difference in LC rates between IMRT and conventional RT [13]. 2- and 5-year LC rates were 62 and 58 %, respectively. However, the complication rate was significantly different with fewer complications in IMRT arm. In 2010, Dirix et al. reported 2-year LC and OS 76 and 89 %, respectively, with postoperative IMRT [19]. Madani et al. found 5-year LC and OS rates of 70.7 and 58.5 %, respectively, in 105 patients more than half of whom had ethmoid sinus tumors [20]. Also in 2012, Duprez et al. showed 5-year LC and OS as 59 and 52 %, respectively [21]. Claus et al. reported their IMRT experience in 62 patients with sinonasal cancers following R0 resection [22]. With PTV doses of 60–70 Gy, they found that none of the patients with cribriform plate invasion were locally controlled. However, 5-year actuarial LC rate was 84 % in patients without cribriform plate invasion.

Stereotactic body radiotherapy (SBRT) may also be an alternative option particularly to spare optic pathway structures. Ozyigit et al. published their experience on 27 patients with paranasal sinus or nasal cavity tumors whom they treated with CyberKnife® (Accuray, Sunnyvale, CA, USA) [23]. Six patients received RT for recurrence. Median dose was 31 Gy in median 5 fractions. They reported local relapse-free rates of 76 % for 21.4 months in median. Overall survival rates in 1 and 2 years were 95.2 and 77.1 %, respectively, with acceptable complication rates.

Chemotherapy

The role of chemotherapy (CT) in nasal cavity and paranasal cancers is limited. Neoadjuvant CT may be used for reducing the tumor size in order to assist surgery in terms of removal of the tumor with less morbidity and also to lend a hand to radiation oncologists in terms of decreasing normal tissue toxicity. In locally advanced tumors, the LC rates are better with concurrent CRT compared to neoadjuvant CT. For unresectable tumors, and medically inoperable patients, CRT is an option.

3   Target Volume Determination and Delineation Guidelines

Gross Tumor Volume (GTV)

GTV should include the gross tumor and involved lymph nodes detected by clinical and endoscopic examination, CT, MRI, PET/CT, and intraoperative findings, if operated. GTV is divided into two: GTVp defines the primary tumor, and GTVn defines the involved lymph nodes. In postoperative cases, GTV is not stated as it is assumed that the primary lesion or grossly involved lymph nodes are removed.

Following structures should be evaluated carefully whether they are involved in case of specific tumors:

- Maxillary Sinus:
  - Anteriorly:
    Is subcutaneous tissue involved?
    Is there extension to the skin of cheek (leading to destruction in zygomatic arch)?
  - Laterally:
    Is the pterygoid fossa involved?
    Is there tumor extension to the sphenoid sinuses?
  - Medially:
    Are the middle meatus and the nasal septum intact?
  - Posteriorly:
    Is the posterior wall intact?
    Are the pterygoid plates, pterygopalatine fossa and muscles involved?
    Is there extension into the infratemporal fossa (through the cribriform plate)?
    Are the clivus and C1 vertebra involved?
    Does the tumor extend to the nasopharynx?
  - Superiorly:
    Are the floor and medial wall of the orbit intact?
    Is the ethmoid sinus involved?
    Is the cribriform plate intact?
  - Inferiorly:
    Is the hard palate involved?
    Is there loosening of the first and second molar teeth (which points out invasion of maxilla)?
- Ethmoid Sinus:
  - Anteriorly:
    Is frontal sinus involved?
    Is there extension to the anterior orbit?
    Is the anterior cranial fossa intact?
    Does the tumor extend to the maxillary sinus?
    Is the palate involved?
  - Laterally:
    Are the orbital medial wall and floor involved?
    Does the tumor extend to the nasal cavity or the orbital rectus muscle?
  - Medially:
    Is contralateral ethmoid sinus intact?
  - Posteriorly:
    Is the sphenoid sinus involved?
    Are the pterygoid plates intact?
    Is there extension into the orbital apex, brain, middle cranial fossa, or clivus?
    Is the cranial nerve (CN) I (olfactory) involved?
    Is the dura involved?
    Does the tumor extend to the nasopharynx?
  - Superiorly:
    Is the cribriform plate intact?

– Inferiorly:
   Is the maxillary sinus involved?
   Is there extension to the nasal cavity?
   Does the tumor extend to the hard palate?

Clinical Target Volume (CTV)

Three CTVs are defined based on risk definitions. CTV1 covers the primary tumor bed with a 1–1.5 cm margin given circumferentially around the GTV.

- *CTV1* for the lymph nodes is the high-risk regions with a gross lymph node, or levels with positive lymph nodes and extracapsular extension (ECE) following lymph node dissection.
- *CTV2* covers the entire operative bed as it is the region of high risk for subclinical disease and potential routes of spread. If the ethmoid sinus or olfactory region is involved, the cribriform plate is also included. For paranasal sinus tumors, CTV2 includes all other sinuses, if explored during surgery. If orbital exenteration was performed because of orbital invasion, the bony orbit is also delineated. In case of craniofacial resection, the frontal graft should also be included. CTV2 for the lymph nodes should include ipsilateral submandibular and subdigastric lymph nodes for squamous cell and poorly or undifferentiated carcinomas. The lower neck should be contoured in case of invasion of the palate, nasopharynx, skin of the cheek or the anterior nose, or gingiva.
- *CTV3* is the low-risk regions for subclinical disease. In case of perineural invasion (PNI), a CTV3 is delineated in order to encompass the whole tract of the submandibular nerve to the skull base. In all adenoid cystic histologies, local nerve pathway to the skull base should be delineated, as these tumors are highly neurotrophic.

In patients who received neoadjuvant CT, CTV is defined depending on the pre-chemotherapy volumes.

Planning Target Volume (PTV)

A margin of 3–5 mm is added in all directions. However, it may be minimized to 1 mm or may even be omitted in areas adjacent to critical structures such as the optic nerves.

Case Contouring

Delineation of target volumes of T4bN2bM0 maxillary sinus carcinoma is shown in Figs. 4.2 and 4.3a–c.

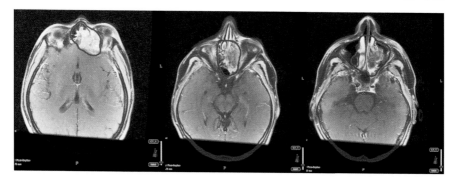

Fig. 4.2 Fused MR simulation CT images of GTV for T4bN2bM0 maxillary sinus cancer

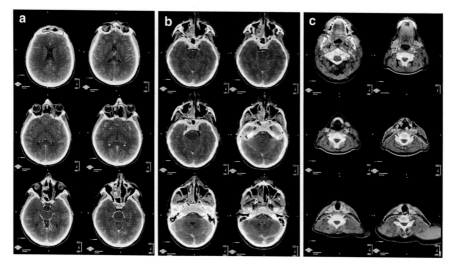

Fig. 4.3 (**a–c**) Delineation of target and normal volumes for T4bN2bM0 maxillary sinus cancer. (Surgical bed: $CTVp_{60Gy}$ *red line*; bilateral levels I, II, and RPLN: $CTVn_{60Gy}$ *blue line*; bilateral levels III, IV, and V: $CTVn_{54Gy}$ *orange*)

4   Treatment Planning

- *Guidelines for Target Volume Doses*: Guidelines for target volume doses are summarized in Table 4.1.
- *Guidelines for Normal Tissue Constraints*: Guidelines for normal tissue constraints are summarized in Table 4.2.
- *Treatment Planning Assessment* (Figs. 4.4 and 4.5)
    - *Step 1*: Check whether the targets are adequately covered: All plans should be normalized to at least 95 % of the volume of PTV70 which is covered by the

Table 4.1 Guidelines for target volume doses

TNM	CTV1 (70 Gy/33–35 fr)	CTV2 (59.4–63 Gy/33–35 fr)	CTV3 (54–56 Gy/33–35 fr)
T1–2 N0	GTVp	–	–
T3–4 N0	GTVp	1–1.5 cm	Ipsilateral I–II, RPLN
Tany N+	GTVp, GTVn	Ipsilateral adjacent lymph nodes (the one level above, and the one level below)	Remaining lymph nodes (ipsilateral, contralateral, and RPLN for advanced tumors)

RPLN retropharyngeal lymph nodes

Table 4.2 Guidelines for normal tissue constraints

Structure	Constraints
Brain	Mean <50 Gy
	For large volumes, <30 Gy
Brain stem	Maximum <54 Gy (no more than 1 % to exceed 60 Gy)
Spinal cord	Maximum <45 Gy (no more than 1 % to exceed 50 Gy)
Eyes	Maximum <50 Gy
Lenses	Maximum <10 Gy, try to achieve <5 Gy (as low as possible)
Optic nerves	<50 Gy
	Maximum <54 Gy
Optic chiasm	<50 Gy
	Maximum <54 Gy
Parotid glands	Mean of one gland <26 Gy
	50 % volume of one gland <30 Gy
	20 cc of both glands <20 Gy
Submandibular and sublingual glands	As low as possible
Each cochlea	Volume receiving 55 Gy <5 %
Mandibula and temporomandibular joint	Maximum <70 Gy (no more than 1 cc to exceed 75 Gy)
Oral cavity (excluding PTVs)	Mean <30–40 Gy
	No hot points receiving >60 Gy in oral cavity region
Lips	Mean <20 Gy
	Maximum <30 Gy
Esophagus, postcricoid pharynx	Mean <45 Gy
Glottic larynx	Mean <45 Gy
Brachial plexus	Maximum <66 Gy

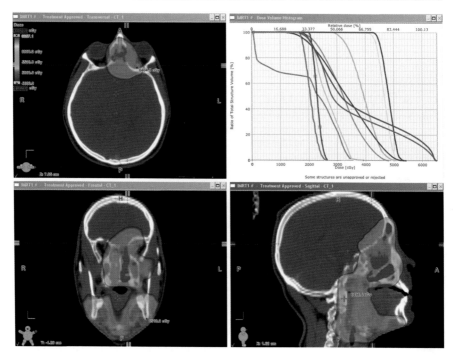

Fig. 4.4 Sagittal, coronal, and axial sections of IMRT plan for T4bN2bM0 maxillary sinus cancer

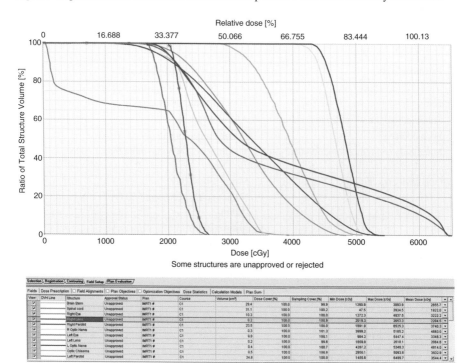

Fig. 4.5 Dose volume histogram for T4bN2bM0 maxillary sinus cancer

70 Gy isodose surface and 99 % of PTV70 needs to be at or above 65.1 Gy. It is confusing to evaluate all PTV DVHs, and one may end up slight underdosing of PTV2 and PTV3 when a uniform 3 mm margin is added, which is generally 80 % coverage of PTV2 and PTV3 mostly due to parotid or critical structure sparing. However, if your nodal CTVs are relatively generous including some muscle outside of the nodal fat plane, much of the setup error is "built in" to the CTV contour drawn, so some physicians only evaluate CTV2 and CTV3 by looking at dose distributions on the treatment plan and not PTV DVH. It is very important to evaluate the DVH of PTV1, because a very tight margin on CTV1 could result in underdosing of gross disease due to daily setup error. Be careful to ensure that PTV1 should receive at least >90 % of prescribed dose.

- – *Step 2*: Check whether there is a large hot spot: No more than 20 % of PTV70 is at or above 77 Gy, and no more than 5 % of PTV70 is at or above 80 Gy.
- – *Step 3*: Check whether the normal tissue constraints are met.
- – *Step 4*: Check whether the hot/cold spots exist in the wrong place (slide by slide looking at isodose distribution): The hot spots need to be arranged in the GTV, and it is necessary to make sure that the hot spot is not on a nerve in the CTV.
- *Case Plan*: The case presented here was treated with IMRT as shown in Fig. 4.6a–c. Surgical bed as $CTVp_{60Gy}$ was prescribed 60 Gy; bilateral levels I, II, and RPLN were irradiated as $CTVn_{60Gy}$ and received 60 Gy; bilateral levels III, IV, and V as $CTVn_{54Gy}$ received 54 Gy.
- *Treatment Algorithm*

Nasal Cavity and Ethmoid Sinus
T1–2, N0, M0
Surgery (in case of close or+surgical margin or PNI add adjuvant RT)
RT
T3–4, N0, M0
If resectable, surgery+adjuvant RT
If unresectable, RT with or without concurrent cisplatin 100 mg/m^2 on days 1, 22, and 43 (or cisplatin 40 mg/m^2/week or carboplatin 100 mg/m^2 on days 1, 8, 15, 22, 29, and 36 or cetuximab 250 mg/m^2/week after a loading dose of 400 mg/m^2 1 week before RT)
Any T, ≥N1, M0
Surgery+adjuvant RT with or without concurrent cisplatin 100 mg/m^2 on days 1, 22, and 43 (or cisplatin 40 mg/m^2/week or carboplatin 100 mg/m^2 on days 1, 8, 15, 22, 29, and 36 or cetuximab 250 mg/m^2/week after a loading dose of 400 mg/m^2 1 week before RT)
CRT (concurrent cisplatin 100 mg/m^2 on days 1, 22, and 43) (or cisplatin 40 mg/m^2/week or carboplatin 100 mg/m^2 on days 1, 8, 15, 22, 29, and 36 or cetuximab 250 mg/m^2/week after a loading dose of 400 mg/m^2 1 week before RT)
Maxillary Sinus
T1–2, N0, M0
Surgery (in case of close or+surgical margin, PNI, or adenoid cystic histology add adjuvant RT)
T3–4, N0, M0
If resectable, surgery+adjuvant RT with or without concurrent cisplatin 100 mg/m^2 on days 1, 22, and 43 (or cisplatin 40 mg/m^2/week or carboplatin 100 mg/m^2 on days 1, 8, 15, 22, 29, and 36 or cetuximab 250 mg/m^2/week after a loading dose of 400 mg/m^2 1 week before RT)

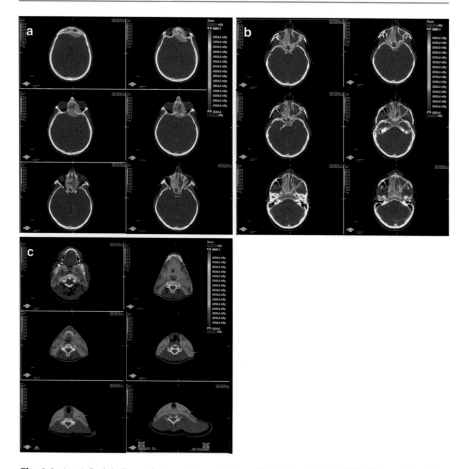

Fig. 4.6 (a–c) Serial slices of dose color wash from IMRT plan for T4bN2bM0 maxillary sinus cancer

---

If unresectable, RT/CRT (concurrent cisplatin 100 mg/m^2 on days 1, 22, and 43) (or cisplatin 40 mg/m^2/week or carboplatin 100 mg/m^2 on days 1, 8, 15, 22, 29, and 36 or cetuximab 250 mg/m^2/week after a loading dose of 400 mg/m^2 1 week before RT)

Any T, ≥N1, M0

Surgery (with neck dissection)+adjuvant RT with or without concurrent cisplatin 100 mg/m^2 on days 1, 22, and 43) (or cisplatin 40 mg/m^2/week or carboplatin 100 mg/m^2 on days 1, 8, 15, 22, 29, and 36 or cetuximab 250 mg/m^2/week after a loading dose of 400 mg/m^2 1 week before RT)

CRT (concurrent cisplatin 100 mg/m^2 on days 1, 22, and 43) (or cisplatin 40 mg/m^2/week or carboplatin 100 mg/m^2 on days 1, 8, 15, 22, 29, and 36 or cetuximab 250 mg/m^2/week after a loading dose of 400 mg/m^2 1 week before RT)

- *Follow-Up*: Every 3 months for the first 2 years, every 4 months for year 3, every 6 months for years 4–5, and then annually. Complete remission through clinical and endoscopic examination and imaging studies is necessary. Distinguish viable residual or slowly regressing tumor, or post-therapy changes by MRI and PET/CT.

References

1. Roush GC (1979) Epidemiology of cancer of the nose and paranasal sinuses: current concepts. Head Neck Surg 2(1):3–11
2. Acheson ED et al (1968) Nasal cancer in woodworkers in the furniture industry. Br Med J 2(5605):587–96
3. Acheson ED, Hadfield EH, Macbeth RG (1967) Carcinoma of the nasal cavity and accessory sinuses in woodworkers. Lancet 1(7485):311–2
4. Klintenberg C et al (1984) Adenocarcinoma of the ethmoid sinuses. A review of 28 cases with special reference to wood dust exposure. Cancer 54(3):482–8
5. Schwaab G, Julieron M, Janot F (1997) Epidemiology of cancers of the nasal cavities and paranasal sinuses. Neurochirurgie 43(2):61–3
6. Torjussen W, Solberg LA, Hogetveit AC (1979) Histopathological changes of the nasal mucosa in active and retired nickel workers. Br J Cancer 40(4):568–80
7. Duthoy W et al (2005) Postoperative intensity-modulated radiotherapy in sinonasal carcinoma: clinical results in 39 patients. Cancer 104(1):71–82
8. Langendijk JA et al (2004) Radiotherapy of squamous cell carcinoma of the nasal vestibule. Int J Radiat Oncol Biol Phys 59(5):1319–25
9. Le QT et al (2000) Lymph node metastasis in maxillary sinus carcinoma. Int J Radiat Oncol Biol Phys 46(3):541–9
10. Mendenhall WM et al (2006) Sinonasal undifferentiated carcinoma. Am J Clin Oncol 29(1):27–31
11. Mendenhall WM et al (1999) Squamous cell carcinoma of the nasal vestibule. Head Neck 21(5):385–93
12. Mazeron JJ et al (1988) Radiation therapy of carcinomas of the skin of nose and nasal vestibule: a report of 1676 cases by the Groupe Europeen de Curietherapie. Radiother Oncol 13(3):165–73
13. Daly ME et al (2007) Intensity-modulated radiation therapy for malignancies of the nasal cavity and paranasal sinuses. Int J Radiat Oncol Biol Phys 67(1):151–7
14. Ang KK et al (1992) Carcinomas of the nasal cavity. Radiother Oncol 24(3):163–8
15. Waldron JN et al (1998) Ethmoid sinus cancer: twenty-nine cases managed with primary radiation therapy. Int J Radiat Oncol Biol Phys 41(2):361–9
16. Choussy O et al (2008) Adenocarcinoma of Ethmoid: a GETTEC retrospective multicenter study of 418 cases. Laryngoscope 118(3):437–43
17. Blanco AI et al (2004) Carcinoma of paranasal sinuses: long-term outcomes with radiotherapy. Int J Radiat Oncol Biol Phys 59(1):51–8
18. Parsons JT et al (1994) Radiation optic neuropathy after megavoltage external-beam irradiation: analysis of time-dose factors. Int J Radiat Oncol Biol Phys 30(4):755–63
19. Dirix P et al (2010) Intensity-modulated radiotherapy for sinonasal cancer: improved outcome compared to conventional radiotherapy. Int J Radiat Oncol Biol Phys 78(4):998–1004
20. Madani I et al (2009) Intensity-modulated radiotherapy for sinonasal tumors: Ghent University Hospital update. Int J Radiat Oncol Biol Phys 73(2):424–32
21. Duprez F et al (2012) IMRT for sinonasal tumors minimizes severe late ocular toxicity and preserves disease control and survival. Int J Radiat Oncol Biol Phys 83(1):252–9
22. Claus F et al (2002) Short term toxicity profile for 32 sinonasal cancer patients treated with IMRT. Can we avoid dry eye syndrome? Radiother Oncol 64(2):205–8
23. Ozyigit G et al (2014) Robotic stereotactic radiosurgery in patients with nasal cavity and paranasal sinus tumors. Technol Cancer Res Treat 13(5):409–13

Oral Cavity

5

Sezin Yuce Sari, Gokhan Ozyigit, Melis Gultekin,
Gozde Yazici, Pervin Hurmuz, Mustafa Cengiz,
and Murat Beyzadeoglu

Overview

Epidemiology

The oral cavity tumors are composed of the tumors of the lips (most common), oral tongue (anterior two thirds of tongue) (second most common), hard palate, buccal mucosa, retromolar trigone, alveolar ridge, and floor of mouth. Oral cavity cancers constitute approximately 3 % of all cancers and 30 % of all head and neck cancers in the USA [1]. It is mostly seen in males of older age. There is a strong correlation between oral cavity cancers and smoking and alcohol consumption, both independently and synergistically [2–5]. Tongue cancers have a trend of increasing in incidence in the young population who are nonsmokers and nondrinkers, which may be due to genetic instability [6, 7]. Ultraviolet radiation has shown to be one of the causes of lip cancer [8]. Certain viruses, namely, herpes simplex virus (HSV) and human papillomavirus (HPV) (particularly HPV-6 and HPV-16), disorders such as Plummer-Vinson syndrome (iron-deficiency anemia, hypopharyngeal webs, and dysphagia), xeroderma pigmentosum, ataxia telangiectasia, Bloom syndrome, and Fanconi's anemia are also associated with oral cavity cancers [9–12]. Patients with oral cavity cancer were proved to be at increased risk for a secondary primary head and neck and esophagus cancer, which affect the prognosis negatively [13, 14].

S.Y. Sari, MD (✉) • G. Ozyigit, MD • M. Gultekin, MD • G. Yazici, MD
P. Hurmuz, MD • M. Cengiz, MD
Department of Radiation Oncology, Hacettepe University, Faculty of Medicine,
Sihhiye, Ankara, Turkey
e-mail: sezin_yuce@hotmail.com

M. Beyzadeoglu, MD
Department of Radiation Oncology, Gulhane Military Medical School, Etlik, Ankara, Turkey

© Springer International Publishing Switzerland 2015
M. Beyzadeoglu et al. (eds.), *Radiation Therapy for Head and Neck Cancers:
A Case-Based Review*, DOI 10.1007/978-3-319-10413-3_5

Pathological and Biological Features

There are premalignant lesions for the development of oral cavity cancers, such as leukoplakia and erythroplakia. These lesions were shown to have loss of heterozygosity at 3p14 and 9p21 locations where the mutations at 17p13 lead to malignant transformation. Approximately 95 % of the malignant tumors are squamous cell carcinoma and its variants (i.e., basaloid, verrucous) [15]. Basaloid type has a poor prognosis as it is mostly diagnosed in advanced or metastatic stage [16], whereas verrucous carcinoma has favorable prognosis with a low rate of distant metastases [17]. Rare histologic subtypes include adenocarcinoma, melanoma, lymphoma, sarcoma, Kaposi's sarcoma, and ameloblastoma.

Definitive Therapy

Early-stage tumors are treated with a single modality of surgery or radiotherapy with similar local control rates. Locally advanced tumors generally need combined treatment modalities.

Adjuvant Therapy

Adjuvant radiotherapy is recommended in high-risk patients with advanced tumor, positive lymph nodes, and perineural invasion. Adjuvant concomitant chemoradiotherapy is indicated for patients with positive surgical margins and extracapsular extension.

1   Case Presentation

Case 1

A 62-year-old female with no history of cigarette smoking or alcohol use was admitted to the hospital with a complaint of a wound in the right part of oral tongue for nearly 6 months. She did not have any additional symptoms. She had diabetes type II, and it was under control with oral antidiabetic use.

Her physical and endoscopic examination revealed a 4×4 cm ulserovegetative lesion extending from the right lateral part of the oral tongue to the tonsillar region posteriorly. The lesion invaded the base of the tongue, the right tonsil, and the floor of mouth at the right side. Vallecula, nasopharynx, larynx, and hypopharynx were normal. There were no palpable lymphadenopathies in the neck.

The MRI revealed a 42×25×25 mm lesion on the right side of oral tongue (Fig. 5.1). It crossed the midline through the medial genioglossus muscle superiorly and invaded the geniohyoid muscle inferiorly and mylohyoid and hyoglossus muscles posteriorly. An irregular signal intensity was defined at the anterior and lateral parts of palatopharyngeal muscle. The margin between stylopharyngeal and medial pterygoid muscles was erased. Right parts of the uvula and the palatine tonsil were asymmetrical compared to the left one. The pharyngopalatine muscle was thicker at

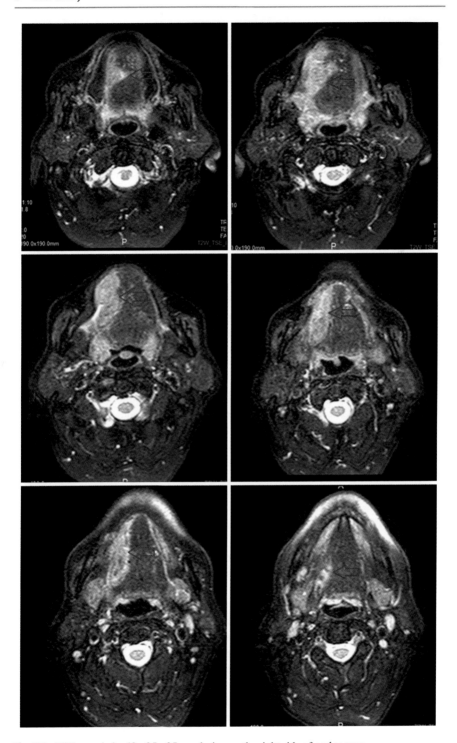

Fig. 5.1 MRI revealed a 42×25×25 mm lesion on the right side of oral tongue

the right. Pathologic lymph nodes were detected in the submental, bilateral submandibular, superior jugular, posterior cervical, suboccipital, and bilateral intraparotid regions.

The biopsy from the lesion in the tongue revealed well-differentiated squamous cell carcinoma (SCC). Right mandibulectomy and right selective neck dissection (levels I–IV) were performed with reconstruction using the major pectoral muscle. The pathology revealed moderately differentiated SCC. The tumor was $2.5 \times 1.2 \times 1.2$ cm. There was diffuse perineural invasion (PNI). Surgical margins were negative, and 35 dissected lymph nodes were free of tumor.

The patient was staged as T2N0M0 oral tongue cancer.

Case 2

A 51-year-old male admitted to the hospital with an unhealing wound in the buccal mucosa of his left cheek.

His physical and endoscopic examination revealed a 1.5×1.5 cm lesion in the left buccal mucosa. There was no invasion in the nasopharynx, hard palate, oropharynx, or larynx. No lymph nodes were palpated.

The MRI detected an $18 \times 11 \times 15$ mm lesion extending from the left buccal mucosa to left cheek fat pad (Fig. 5.2). It was located posterior to the maxilla and at the level of retromolar region. There were reactive lymph nodes, <1 cm in size in left level IA and bilateral level II.

The incisional biopsy from mucosal lesion revealed squamous cell carcinoma (SCC). He underwent wide local excision of the primary and left level I–V neck dissection. The pathologic evaluation was reported as moderately differentiated SCC. The tumor was $1.7 \times 1.5 \times 0.4$ cm. Out of 37 dissected lymph nodes, 2 were metastatic and had extracapsular extension (ECE).

He was staged as T1N2bM0 buccal mucosa cancer.

2   Evidence-Based Treatment Approaches

Transoral or transcervical surgery is generally the first choice for early stage lesions [17]. More aggressive surgeries like mandibulectomy are performed when the lesion cannot be reached by these techniques or when there is bone invasion.

In early lesions of the lip, oral tongue, and floor of the mouth, radiotherapy (RT) and surgery are equivalent in terms of local control (LC) [18]. Historical series reported increased LC rates with the use of brachytherapy (BRT) either alone or in combination with external beam radiotherapy (EBRT) [19, 20]. Different authors reported LC rates that ranged from 70 to 96 % for T1 and T2 tumors [21–24].

Combined treatment modalities are preferred for locally advanced tumors [20, 25–27]. In case of mandibular invasion, definitive RT is contraindicated as LC results are poor with high risk of osteoradionecrosis. Postoperative RT is often preferred over preoperative RT to prevent a delay in surgery, to decrease the risk of wound

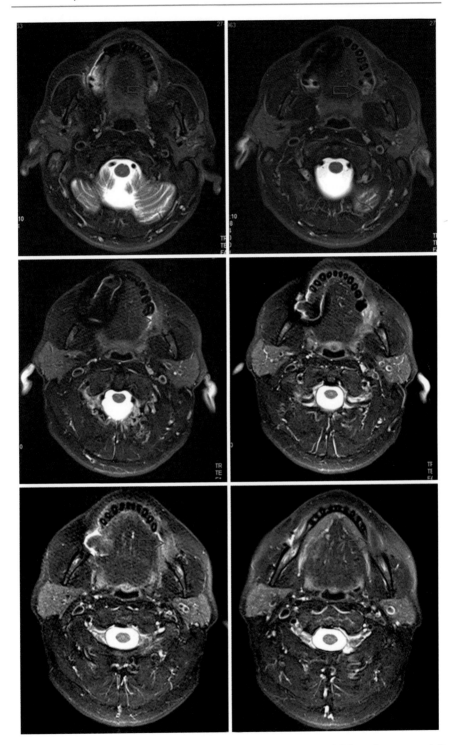

Fig. 5.2 MRI showing an $18 \times 11 \times 15$ mm lesion extending from the left buccal mucosa to left cheek fat pad, located posterior to the maxilla, and at the level of retromolar region

complications, and to provide complete histologic evaluation. The disadvantage of postoperative RT is regional hypoxia which decreases the effectiveness of RT.

Postoperative RT is indicated in case of advanced T stage, suspected mandibular invasion, perineural invasion (PNI), close or positive surgical margins, multiple lymph node positivity, and/or extracapsular extension (ECE).

Neoadjuvant or adjuvant chemotherapy (CT), containing cis-platinum and 5-FU, was reported to have no impact on survival [28, 29]. However, adding CT concurrently to RT resulted in increased LC and overall survival (OS) rates [30].

Two prospective randomized trials investigated CRT after surgery in high-risk patients [31, 32]. The RTOG 9501 showed that in patients with positive surgical margins, two or more positive lymph nodes, or ECE, postoperative CRT increased LRC and disease-free survival (DFS) at the cost of increased toxicity but had no impact on OS. In EORTC 22931 study, in addition to these characteristics, stages III–IV, PNI, vascular tumor embolism, and level IV–V lymph node positivity were also evaluated as high-risk features. Besides the increase in LRC, and progression-free survival (PFS), OS was also superior in the CRT arm. In the report which combined these two trials, the only features that benefited from CRT were surgical margin positivity and ECE. Patients with two or more positive lymph nodes had no benefit from CRT, while patients with other high-risk features had a trend. In the 10-year update of RTOG 9501, the benefit in DFS and LC continued in patients with positive margins and ECE, and the long-term toxicity was reported to be similar to the RT alone group.

Buccal Mucosa

Primary surgery is preferred for small, superficial lesions. For deeper lesions (i.e. T2) or if there is commissure involvement, RT provides better results in terms of function and cosmesis, without any decline in cure rates. For more advanced lesions, radical surgery and adjuvant RT are indicated.

Oral Tongue

For small T1–2 lesions, RT yields better cosmetic and functional results and has similar LC rates compared to surgery. If floor of mouth is involved, partial glossectomy and partial mandibulectomy with radical neck dissection are performed. RT may be an alternative for patients who refuse surgery. Adjuvant RT is indicated in patients with locally advanced tumors, close or positive surgical margins, and PNI.

Floor of the Mouth

Surgery and RT yield comparable results in small, superficial tumors. In case of mandibular invasion, surgery should be preferred. For more advanced lesions (with invasion of bone or adjacent muscles), adjuvant RT is indicated.

Management of the Neck

Small, superficial (depth <2 mm) tumors with negative surgical margins do not require elective neck treatment (in case the patient is clinically node negative). In oral tongue and floor of the mouth tumors deeper than 2 mm, and in all tumors with perineural or perilymphatic invasion, the neck should be treated either with surgical dissection or by RT. Following neck dissection, if there is 1 positive lymph node without ECE, RT to the neck is not recommended [33]. If there are more than 1 positive lymph nodes (particularly at more than one nodal station), or ECE, the neck should be irradiated.

There are limited studies with IMRT on oral cavity tumors. Chao et al. from Washington University reported their initial results of 15 patients with oral cavity cancers whom they treated with IMRT [34]. Locoregional recurrence and distant metastasis were observed in 5 and 1 patients, respectively. There was no grade 3 or higher late toxicity. Similarly, Claus et al. treated 8 patients with oral cavity cancers via IMRT and observed no serious late toxicity, except for 1 patient who had mandibular osteoradionecrosis [35].

3   Target Volume Determination and Delineation Guidelines

Gross Tumor Volume (GTV)

GTV should include the gross tumor and involved lymph nodes detected by clinical examination, CT, MRI, PET/CT, and intraoperative findings, if operated. GTV is divided into two; GTVp defines the primary tumor, and GTVn defines the involved lymph nodes. In postoperative cases without residual tumor, GTV is not stated as it is assumed that no tumor or grossly involved lymph nodes are left.

Following structures should be evaluated carefully whether they are involved in oral tongue tumors:

- Anteriorly:
  Is the skin of face involved?
- Laterally:
  Is the skin of face involved?
  Is the cortical bone of the mandible destructed?
- Posteriorly:
  Are the pterygoid plates involved?
  Is there extension into the masticator space?
  Is the carotid artery involved?
- Superiorly:
  Is the maxillary sinus intact?
  Is the hard palate involved?
  Is the skull base destructed?

- Inferiorly:
  Is the floor of mouth involved?
  Is there extension to deep extrinsic muscles (genioglossus, hyoglossus, palatoglossus, and styloglossus)?

Clinical Target Volume (CTV)

Three CTVs are defined based on risk definitions.

- *CTV1* covers the primary tumor bed with a 0.5–2 cm margin given circumferentially around the GTV. CTV1 for the lymph nodes is the high-risk regions with a gross lymph node or, following lymph node dissection, levels with positive lymph nodes and extracapsular extension.
- *CTV2* covers the entire operative bed as it is the region of high risk for subclinical disease and potential routes of spread, along with the high-risk regions adjacent to it. Certain routes of spread are defined for particular locations. These are sublingual gland, midline genioglossus and geniohyoid muscles, periosteum, and mandible for floor of mouth cancers; floor of mouth, base of tongue, muscles of tongue, anterior tonsillar pillar, and mandible for oral tongue cancers; underlying muscles, skin, infratemporal fossa, parotid gland, and facial nerve for buccal mucosa cancers; and adjacent buccal mucosa, anterior tonsillar pillar, lower gum, maxilla, and mandible for retromolar trigone. *CTV2* for the lymph nodes is ipsilateral submandibular, subdigastric, and midjugular nodal stations (upper neck). For tumors of the tip of the tongue, and tumors exceeding midline, upper neck should be contoured bilaterally. Periauricular and intraparotid lymph nodes are also delineated for the tumors of the upper lip. Oral cavity tumors with verrucous histology (which are often seen in the buccal mucosa) do not generally require elective neck irradiation as they rarely metastasize to lymph nodes.
- *CTV3* is the low-risk regions of subclinical disease. CTV3 for the lymph nodes include the contralateral upper neck and bilateral lower neck (lower jugular and supraclavicular). Ipsilateral posterior neck and retropharyngeal lymph nodes should also be delineated in the presence of jugular positive lymph nodes.

In patients who received neoadjuvant CT, CTV is defined depending on the pre-chemotherapy volumes.

Planning Target Volume (PTV)

A margin of 3–5 mm is added in all directions; however, it may be minimized to 1 mm in areas adjacent to critical structures.

Case Contouring

Delineation of target volumes for T2N0M0 oral tongue cancer (Case 1) is depicted in Fig. 5.3.

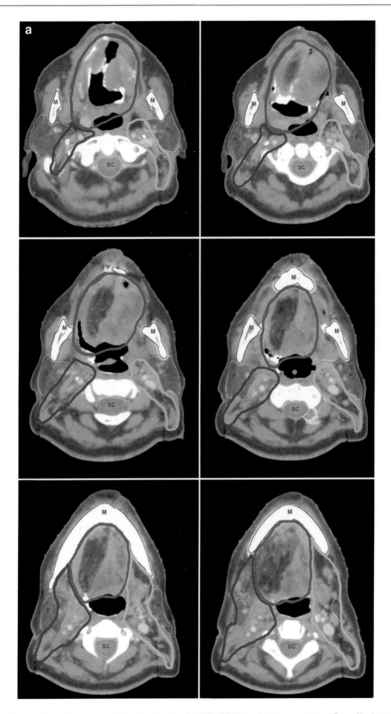

Fig. 5.3 (**a**, **b**) Delineation of target volumes for T2N0M0 oral tongue cancer (Case 1). (surgical bed, CTVp$_{60Gy}$ *magenta*; right neck, CTVn$_{57Gy}$ *red*; left neck, CTVn$_{54Gy}$ *aqua*) (*BS* brain stem, *OC* oral cavity, *M* mandible, *P* parotid gland, *SC* spinal cord, *E* epiglottis, *V* vallecula, *Ps* pyriform sinus, *H* hyoid bone, *IJV* internal jugular vein, *L* larynx, *CA* common carotid artery, *Cr* cricoid cartilage, *TG* thyroid gland, *T* trapezius muscle, *E* esophagus, *TCV* transverse cervical vessels)

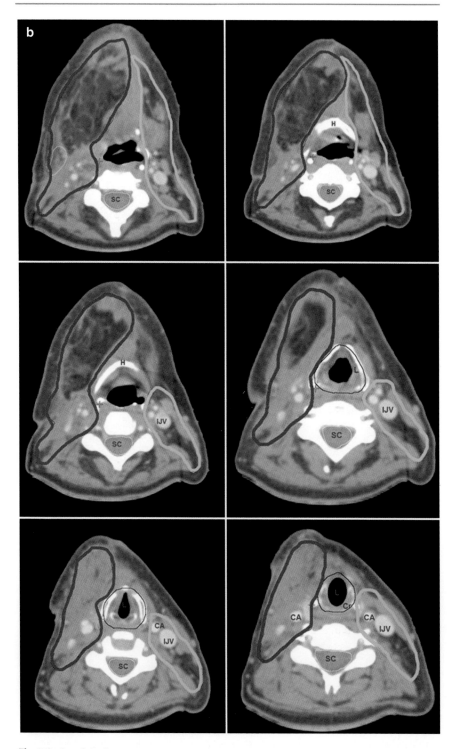

Fig. 5.3 (continued)

Delineation of target volumes for T1N2bM0 buccal mucosa cancer (Case 2) is depicted in Figs. 5.4 and 5.5.

4   Treatment Planning

- *Guidelines for target volume doses*: Guidelines for target volume doses are summarized in Tables 5.1, 5.2, and 5.3.
- *Guidelines for normal tissue constraints*: Guidelines for normal tissue constraints are summarized in Table 5.4.
- *Treatment Planning Assessment* (Figs. 5.6, 5.7, 5.8, and 5.9)
  - *Step 1*: Check whether the targets are adequately covered. All plans should be normalized to at least 95 % of the volume of PTV70 which is covered by the 70 Gy isodose surface and 99 % of PTV70 which needs to be at or above 65.1 Gy. It is confusing to evaluate all PTV DVHs, and one may end up slight underdosing of PTV2 and PTV3 when a uniform 3 mm margin is added, which is generally 80 % coverage of PTV2 and PTV3 mostly due to parotid or critical structure sparing. However, if your nodal CTVs are relatively generous including some muscle outside of the nodal fat plane, much of the setup error is "built in" to the CTV contour drawn, so some physicians only evaluate CTV2 and CTV3 by looking at dose distributions on the treatment plan and not PTV DVH. It is very important to evaluate the DVH of PTV1, because a very tight margin on CTV1 could result in underdosing of gross disease due to daily setup error. Be careful to ensure that PTV1 should receive at least >90 % of prescribed dose.
  - *Step 2*: Check whether there is a large hot spot. No more than 20 % of PTV70 is at or above 77 Gy, and no more than 5 % of PTV70 is at or above 80 Gy.
  - *Step 3*: Check whether the normal tissue constraints are met.
  - *Step 4*: Check whether the hot/cold spots exist in the wrong place (slide by slide looking at isodose distribution). The hot spots need to be arranged in the GTV; it is necessary to make sure that the hot spot is not on a nerve in the CTV.
- *Case Plan 1*: The case 1 (oral tongue cancer) presented here was treated with IMRT as shown in Fig. 5.10. Surgical bed as $CTVp_{60Gy}$ was prescribed 60 Gy, right neck was irradiated as $CTVn_{57Gy}$ and received 57 Gy, and left neck as $CTVn_{54Gy}$ received 54 Gy. Concurrent chemotherapy was not given.
- *Case Plan 2*: The case 2 (buccal mucosa cancer) presented here was treated with IMRT as shown in Fig. 5.11. Right level I and surgical bed as CTV_{60Gy} was prescribed 60 Gy, left level II was irradiated as $CTVn_{64Gy}$ and received 64 Gy, left level II–V was irradiated as $CTVn_{57Gy}$ and received 57 Gy, right levels II, IV, and V as $CTVn_{54Gy}$ received 54 Gy. Concurrent cisplatin was given weekly with a dose of 35 mg/m^2.

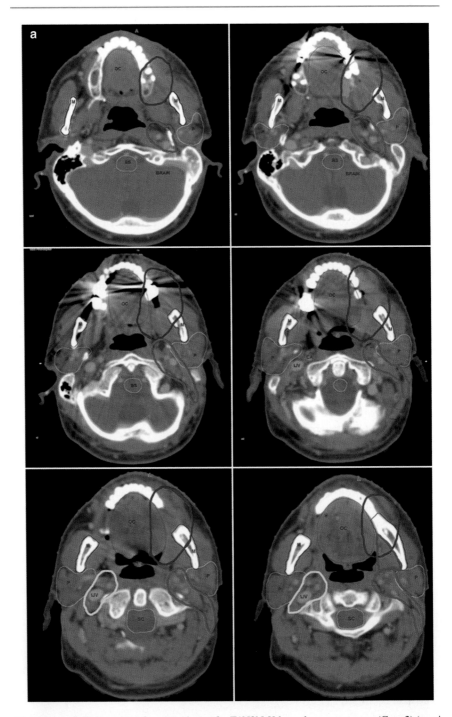

Fig. 5.4 (**a–d**) Delineation of target volumes for T1N2bM0 buccal mucosa cancer (Case 2) (surgical bed and right level I, CTVp$_{60Gy}$ *red*; left level I–V, CTVn$_{57Gy}$ *yellow*; right levels II–V, CTVn$_{54Gy}$ *blue*; right level Ib, CTVn$_{60Gy}$ *blue*; left level II, CTVn$_{64Gy}$ *magenta*) (*M* mandible, *P* parotid gland, *SC* spinal cord, *H* hyoid bone, *IJV* internal jugular vein, *L* larynx, *CA* common carotid artery, *Cr* cricoid cartilage, *OC* oral cavity, *BS* Brain stem, *V* valleculae, *E* Epiglottis, *Ps* pyriform sinus, *TG* thyroid gland, *T* trapezius muscle)

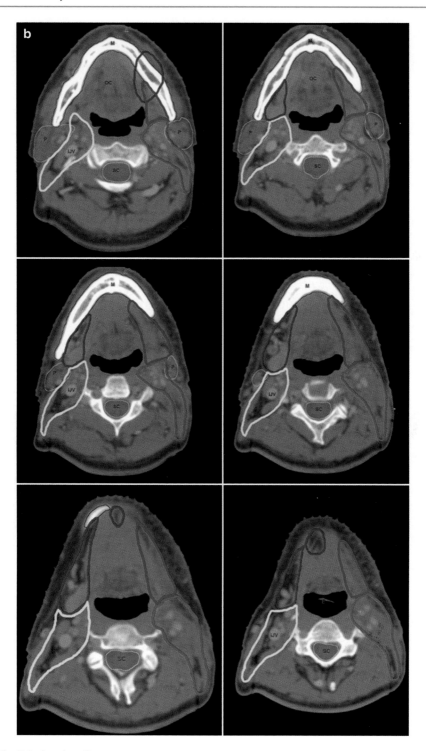

Fig. 5.4 (continued)

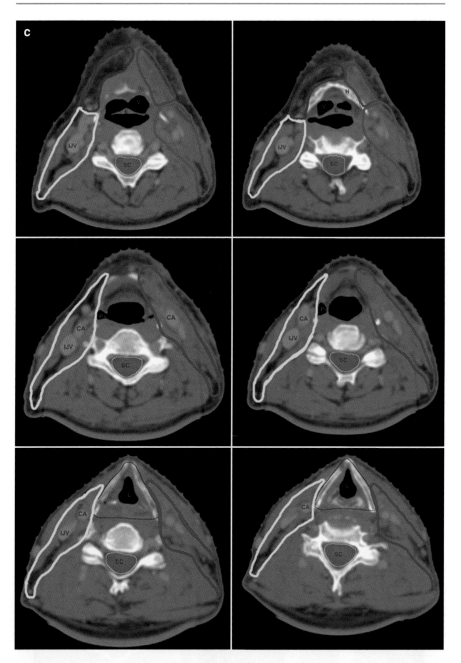

Fig. 5.4 (continued)

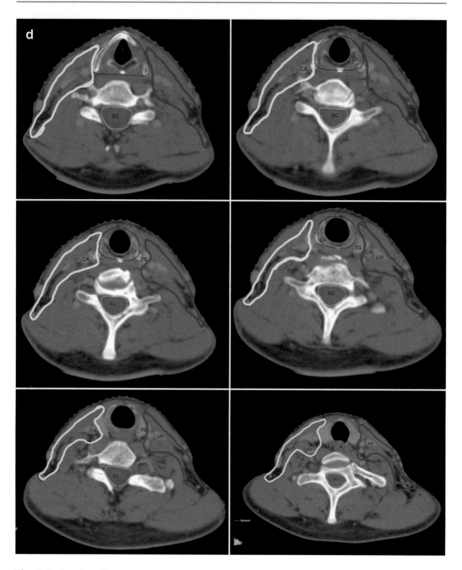

Fig. 5.4 (continued)

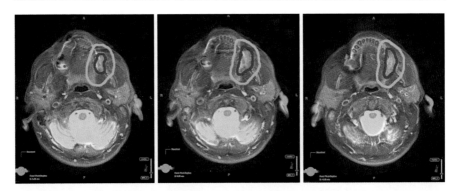

Fig. 5.5 Delineation of GTV and CTV for T1N2bM0 buccal mucosa cancer on fused MRI and BT simulation slices (Case 2)

Table 5.1 Guidelines for target volume doses of lip cancers

TNM	CTV1 66–70 Gy (33–35 fr)	CTV2 59.4–60 Gy (33–35 fr)	CTV3 54 Gy (33–35 fr)
T1–2 N0	GTVp	1.5–2 cm	–
T3–4 N0	GTVp	1.5–2 cm	Ipsilateral I–III
Tany N+	GTVp, GTVn	Ipsilateral adjacent lymph nodes (one level above and one level below)	Remaining lymph nodes (ipsilateral, contralateral, and RP for advanced tumors)

Table 5.2 Guidelines for target volume doses of oral tongue and the floor of mouth cancers

TNM	CTV1 66–70 Gy (33–35 fr)	CTV2 59.4–60 Gy (33–35 fr)	CTV3 54 Gy (33–35 fr)
Tany N0	GTVp	Tumor bed	Bilateral levels I–IV
Tany N+	GTVp, GTVn	Tumor bed and ipsilateral levels I–V (or if contralateral neck + bilateral levels I–V +/– RP)	Contralateral levels I–V (if uninvolved)

Table 5.3 Guidelines for target volume doses retromolar trigone and buccal mucosa cancers

TNM	CTV1 66–70 Gy (33–35 fr)	CTV2 59.4–60 Gy (33–35 fr)	CTV3 54 Gy (33–35 fr)
T1–2 N0	GTVp	Tumor bed	Ipsilateral levels I–IV[a]
T3–4 N0	GTVp	Tumor bed and ipsilateral levels I–IV	GTVn (if not involved; contralateral II–IV or I–V + RP)
Tany N+	GTVp, GTVn	Tumor bed and ipsilateral levels I–V (or if contralateral neck + bilateral levels I–V +/– RP)	GTVn (if not involved; contralateral II–IV or I–V + RP)

RP Retropharyngeal
[a]Based on physician's discretion

Table 5.4 Guidelines for normal tissue constraints

Structure	Constraints
Brain	Mean <50 Gy
	For larger volumes, <30 Gy
Brain stem	Maximum <54 Gy (no more than 1 % to exceed 60 Gy)
Spinal cord	Maximum <45 Gy (no more than 1 % to exceed 50 Gy)
Eyes	Maximum <50 Gy
Lenses	Maximum <10 Gy, try to achieve <5 Gy (as low as possible)
Optic nerves	<50 Gy (maximum <54 Gy)
Optic chiasm	<50 Gy (maximum <54 Gy)
Parotid glands	Mean for one gland <26 Gy or 50 % volume of one gland <30 Gy or 20 cc of both glands <20 Gy
Submandibular and sublingual glands	As low as possible
Each cochlea	Volume receiving 55 Gy <5 %
Mandibula and temporomandibular joint	Maximum <70 Gy (no more than 1 cc to exceed 75 Gy)
Oral cavity (excluding PTVs)	Mean <50 Gy
	No hot points receiving >60 Gy in oral cavity region
Lips (if not in PTV)	Mean <20 Gy
	Maximum <50 Gy
Esophagus, postcricoid pharynx	Mean <45 Gy
Glottic larynx	Mean <45 Gy
Brachial plexus	Maximum <66 Gy

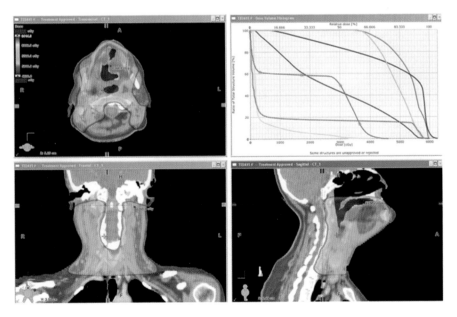

Fig. 5.6 IMRT plan for T2N0M0 oral tongue cancer (Case 1)

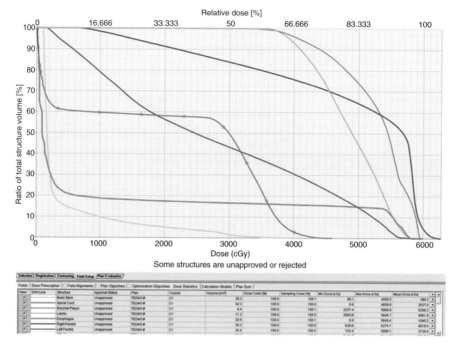

Fig. 5.7 Dose volume histogram (DVH) for normal tissues for T2N0M0 oral tongue cancer (Case 1)

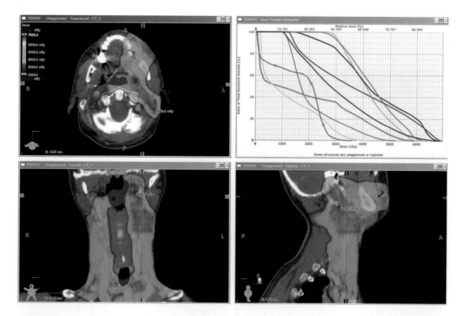

Fig. 5.8 IMRT plan for T1N2bM0 buccal mucosa cancer (Case 2)

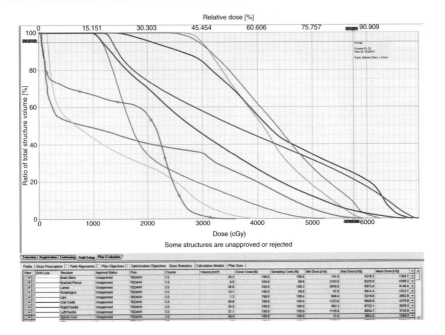

Fig. 5.9 Dose volume histogram (DVH) for normal tissues for T1N2bM0 buccal mucosa cancer (Case 2)

- *Treatment algorithm*

T1–2, N0, M0
RT
Surgery (in case of+surgical margins, add adjuvant RT)
T3–4, ≥N1, M0
Concurrent CRT (concurrent cisplatin 100 mg/m² on days 1, 22, and 43 or cisplatin 40 mg/m²/week or carboplatin 100 mg/m² on days 1, 8, 15, 22, 29, and 36 or cetuximab 250 mg/m²/week after a loading dose of 400 mg/m² 1 week before RT)
Surgery (in case of+surgical margins or extracapsular extension add adjuvant CRT) (concurrent cisplatin 100 mg/m² on days 1, 22, and 43 or cisplatin 40 mg/m²/week or carboplatin 100 mg/m² on days 1, 8, 15, 22, 29, and 36 or cetuximab 250 mg/m²/week after a loading dose of 400 mg/m² 1 week before RT; in case of multiple+lymph nodes, PNI, or lymphovascular space invasion, add adjuvant RT)

- *Follow-up*: Every 3 months for the first 2 years, every 4–6 months for years 3–5, and then annually. Complete remission through clinical and endoscopic examination and imaging studies is necessary. Distinguish viable residual or slowly regressing tumor or post-therapy changes by MRI and PET/CT.

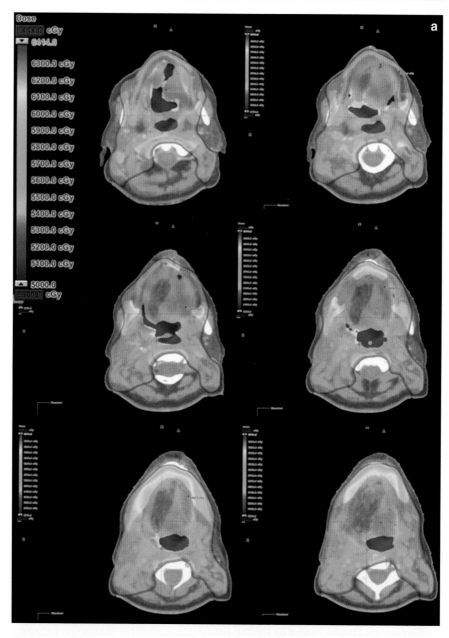

Fig. 5.10 (**a**, **b**) Slice by slice isodose evaluation of IMRT plan for T2N0M0 oral tongue cancer (Case 1)

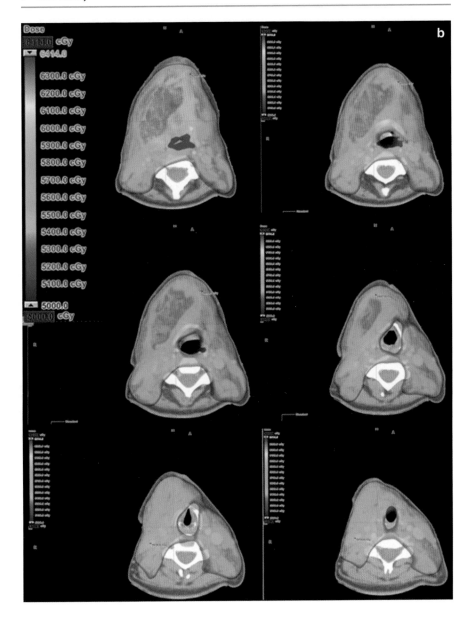

Fig. 5.10 (continued)

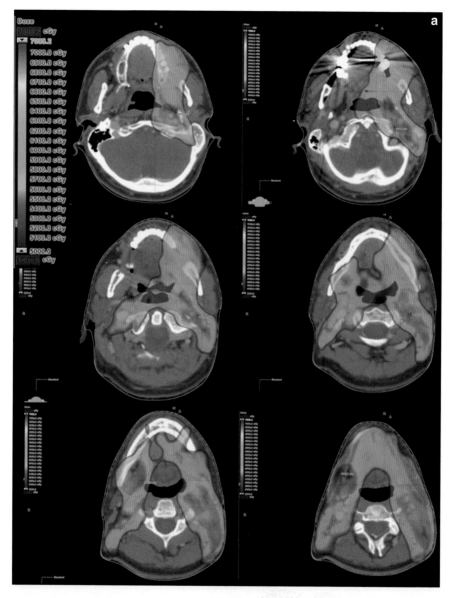

Fig. 5.11 (**a**, **b**) Slice by slice isodose evaluation of IMRT plan for T1N2bM0 buccal mucosa cancer (Case 2)

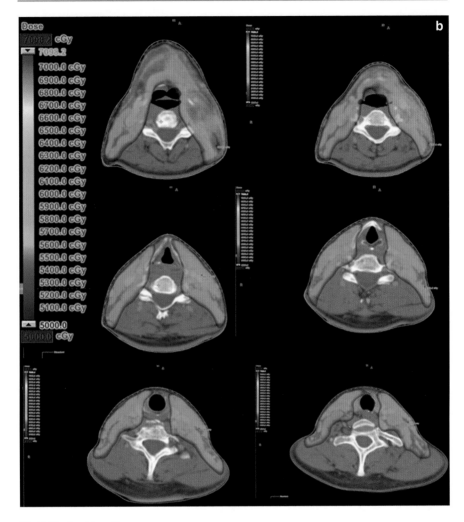

Fig. 5.11 (continued)

References

1. Greenlee RT et al (2000) Cancer statistics, 2000. CA Cancer J Clin 50(1):7–33
2. Dobrossy L (2005) Epidemiology of head and neck cancer: magnitude of the problem. Cancer Metastasis Rev 24(1):9–17
3. Boyle P, Macfarlane GJ, Scully C (1993) Oral cancer: necessity for prevention strategies. Lancet 342(8880):1129
4. Kurumatani N et al (1999) Time trends in the mortality rates for tobacco- and alcohol-related cancers within the oral cavity and pharynx in Japan, 1950–94. J Epidemiol 9(1):46–52
5. Macfarlane GJ et al (1995) Alcohol, tobacco, diet and the risk of oral cancer: a pooled analysis of three case–control studies. Eur J Cancer B Oral Oncol 31B(3):181–187

6. Myers JN et al (2000) Squamous cell carcinoma of the tongue in young adults: increasing incidence and factors that predict treatment outcomes. Otolaryngol Head Neck Surg 122(1):44–51
7. Llewellyn CD, Johnson NW, Warnakulasuriya KA (2001) Risk factors for squamous cell carcinoma of the oral cavity in young people–a comprehensive literature review. Oral Oncol 37(5):401–418
8. Antoniades DZ et al (1995) Squamous cell carcinoma of the lips in a northern Greek population. Evaluation of prognostic factors on 5-year survival rate–I. Eur J Cancer B Oral Oncol 31B(5):333–339
9. Myers E (2003) Cancer of the head and neck. Saunders, Philadelphia
10. Miller CS, Johnstone BM (2001) Human papillomavirus as a risk factor for oral squamous cell carcinoma: a meta-analysis, 1982–1997. Oral Surg Oral Med Oral Pathol Oral Radiol Endod 91(6):622–635
11. Maden C et al (1992) Human papillomaviruses, herpes simplex viruses, and the risk of oral cancer in men. Am J Epidemiol 135(10):1093–1102
12. Prime SS et al (2001) A review of inherited cancer syndromes and their relevance to oral squamous cell carcinoma. Oral Oncol 37(1):1–16
13. Lippman SM, Hong WK (1989) Second malignant tumors in head and neck squamous cell carcinoma: the overshadowing threat for patients with early-stage disease. Int J Radiat Oncol Biol Phys 17(3):691–694
14. Schwartz LH et al (1994) Synchronous and metachronous head and neck carcinomas. Cancer 74(7):1933–1938
15. Green FL et al (2002) AJCC cancer staging manual. Springer, New York
16. Winzenburg SM et al (1998) Basaloid squamous carcinoma: a clinical comparison of two histologic types with poorly differentiated squamous cell carcinoma. Otolaryngol Head Neck Surg 119(5):471–475
17. Chen AY, Myers JN (2001) Cancer of the oral cavity. Dis Mon 47(7):275–361
18. Harrison LB, Fass DE (1990) Radiation therapy for oral cavity cancer. Dent Clin North Am 34(2):205–222
19. Fu KK et al (1976) Time, dose and volume factors in interstitial Radium implants of carcinoma of the oral tongue. Radiology 119(1):209–213
20. Fu KK et al (1976) External and interstitial radiation therapy of carcinoma of the oral tongue. A review of 32 years' experience. AJR Am J Roentgenol 126(1):107–115
21. Dearnaley DP et al (1991) Interstitial irradiation for carcinoma of the tongue and floor of mouth: Royal Marsden Hospital Experience 1970–1986. Radiother Oncol 21(3):183–192
22. Pernot M et al (1995) Evaluation of the importance of systematic neck dissection in carcinoma of the oral cavity treated by brachytherapy alone for the primary lesion (apropos of a series of 346 patients). Bull Cancer Radiother 82(3):311–317
23. Decroix Y, Ghossein NA (1981) Experience of the Curie Institute in treatment of cancer of the mobile tongue: II. Management of the neck nodes. Cancer 47(3):503–508
24. Pernot M et al (1995) Epidermoid carcinomas of the floor of mouth treated by exclusive irradiation: statistical study of a series of 207 cases. Radiother Oncol 35(3):177–185
25. Robertson AG et al (1998) Early closure of a randomized trial: surgery and postoperative radiotherapy versus radiotherapy in the management of intra-oral tumours. Clin Oncol (R Coll Radiol) 10(3):155–160
26. Shah JP, Lydiatt W (1995) Treatment of cancer of the head and neck. CA Cancer J Clin 45(6):352–368
27. Vikram B et al (1980) Elective postoperative radiation therapy in stages III and IV epidermoid carcinoma of the head and neck. Am J Surg 140(4):580–584
28. Licitra L et al (2003) Primary chemotherapy in resectable oral cavity squamous cell cancer: a randomized controlled trial. J Clin Oncol 21(2):327–333
29. Volling P et al (1999) Results of a prospective randomized trial with induction chemotherapy for cancer of the oral cavity and tonsils. HNO 47(10):899–906

30. Mohr C et al (1994) Preoperative radiochemotherapy and radical surgery in comparison with radical surgery alone. A prospective, multicentric, randomized DOSAK study of advanced squamous cell carcinoma of the oral cavity and the oropharynx (a 3-year follow-up). Int J Oral Maxillofac Surg 23(3):140–148
31. Bernier J et al (2004) Postoperative irradiation with or without concomitant chemotherapy for locally advanced head and neck cancer. N Engl J Med 350(19):1945–1952
32. Cooper JS et al (2004) Postoperative concurrent radiotherapy and chemotherapy for high-risk squamous-cell carcinoma of the head and neck. N Engl J Med 350(19):1937–1944
33. Emami B (1998) Oral cavity. In: Brady LW (ed) Principles and practice of radiation oncology. Lippincott-Raven, Philadelphia, pp 981–1002
34. Chao KS et al (2002) Determination and delineation of nodal target volumes for head-and-neck cancer based on patterns of failure in patients receiving definitive and postoperative IMRT. Int J Radiat Oncol Biol Phys 53(5):1174–1184
35. Claus F et al (2002) Intensity modulated radiation therapy for oropharyngeal and oral cavity tumors: clinical use and experience. Oral Oncol 38(6):597–604

Nasopharynx

6

Ugur Selek, Yasemin Bolukbasi, Erkan Topkan, and Gokhan Ozyigit

Overview

Epidemiology

The distribution demonstrates a regional, racial, and gender prevalence (rare in the United States and Western Europe but high in Southern China, Southeast Asia, North Africa, and the Middle East). Individuals with hereditary susceptibility due to early infection with Epstein-Barr virus (EBV) seem to develop NPC when EBV is reactivated. Subgroup of EBV latent proteins, including EBNA-1, LMP-1, and LMP-2 (integral membrane proteins), and the BamHI-A fragment of the EBV genome are expressed in NPC. Several dietary practices are thought to contribute to the high incidence such as cooking of salt-cured food releasing volatile nitrosamines, preserved or fermented foods containing high levels of nitrosamines, and rancid butter and sheep's fat containing butyric acid (a potential EBV activator). Smoking is also associated with NPC.

U. Selek, MD (✉)
Department of Radiation Oncology, Koc University, Faculty of Medicine,
Nisantasi, Istanbul, Turkey

Department of Radiation Oncology, University of Texas MD Anderson Cancer Center,
Houston, TX, USA
e-mail: ugurselek@yahoo.com

Y. Bolukbasi, MD
Department of Radiation Oncology, MD Anderson Radiation Treatment Center,
American Hospital, Nisantasi, Istanbul, Turkey

E. Topkan, MD
Department of Radiation Oncology, Baskent University, Faculty of Medicine, Adana, Turkey

G. Ozyigit, MD
Department of Radiation Oncology, Hacettepe University, Faculty of Medicine,
Sihhiye, Ankara, Turkey

© Springer International Publishing Switzerland 2015   93
M. Beyzadeoglu et al. (eds.), *Radiation Therapy for Head and Neck Cancers:*
A Case-Based Review, DOI 10.1007/978-3-319-10413-3_6

Pathological and Biological Features
WHO classifies three histopathologic types: keratinizing squamous cell carcinoma (sporadic, WHO Type I), nonkeratinizing carcinoma as differentiated (Type II) and undifferentiated (endemic, Type III) forms, and basaloid squamous cell carcinoma. Pretreatment serologic antienzyme rate of Epstein-Barr virus DNase-specific neutralizing antibody segregates TNM classification in nasopharyngeal carcinoma

Definitive Therapy
Radiation therapy is the mainstay of local treatment for stage I, while concurrent chemoradiotherapy is necessary for locoregionally advanced stage (II–IVB) to reduce distant metastasis rate and to improve both local control and overall survival.

Adjuvant Therapy
Benefit of adjuvant chemotherapy is uncertain with substantial toxicity although it is a standard approach in many concurrent chemoradiotherapy regimens.

1   Case Presentation

Thirty-year-old female who was a nonsmoker with no significant past medical history presented with a blocked nose and complain of 6/10 headaches that require the use of Excedrin for relief. She was also complaining of epistaxis periodically as well as coughing blood occasionally. She denied any problems with dysphagia, swallowing, or chewing, as well as any current odynophagia. She has left neck swelling but denied any chest pain, palpitations, or shortness of breath.

Her physical exam revealed normal external ear canals and tympanic membranes with appropriate light reflex. Nasal septum was midline without deviation and was clear to anterior rhinoscopy. She had good dentition. There are no lesions of the gingiva, buccal mucosa, floor of mouth, oral tongue, base of tongue, hard palate, soft palate, tonsillar fossa, or posterior oropharyngeal wall by visualization or palpation. Palate elevates normally. Tongue protrudes normally. There was an approximately 4 cm hardly mobile node in the left upper level II area and was no other palpable adenopathy bilaterally. Cranial nerves II–XII are grossly intact without any facial numbness. The scope was introduced into the left nasal cavity. Clearly seen is a left erythematous nasopharyngeal mass centered on the left fossa of Rosenmuller. It was extending anteriorly to involve the torus and appears to block off the eustachian tube on the left side. It did not extend into the posterior aspect of the nasal cavity. The mass did not medially go past midline and just appeared to be left-sided. The right torus and eustachian tube were free of disease. Superiorly, the mass went up to the roof of the nasopharynx. Inferiorly, it went up to the level of the soft palate. There does not appear to be any posterior pharyngeal wall bulging or lesions. The scope was advanced further. There was no evidence of disease in the oropharynx, larynx, and hypopharynx. Vocal cords were mobile.

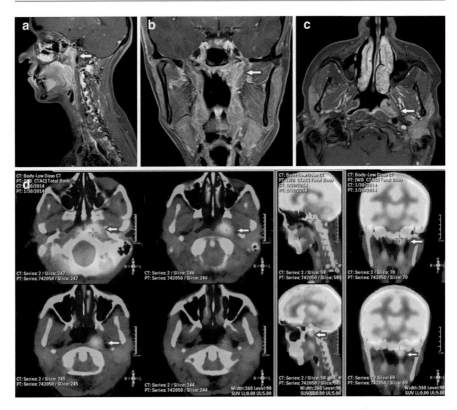

Fig. 6.1 (a–d) MRI sagittal (a) and coronal (b) and axial (c) images and PET-CT (d) display left nasopharyngeal lesion filling the Rosenmuller fossa invading through the pharyngobasilar fascia and infiltrating the cavernous sinus measuring 17×7×26 mm

Both MRI and PET-CT defined left nasopharyngeal lesion filling the Rosenmuller fossa invading through the pharyngobasilar fascia and infiltrating the cavernous sinus measuring 17×7×26 mm (Fig. 6.1a–d). The lesion was minimally extending intracranially through foramen ovale (Fig. 6.2). Both left-sided foramen rotundum and vidian channel were asymmetrically involved with tumor. The imaging also revealed bilateral nodal disease, largest on left level 2 measuring 3.5 cm (Fig. 6.3).

A biopsy was performed from the left nasopharyngeal lesion confirming the undifferentiated nonkeratinizing carcinoma (WHO Type III).

She was staged as T4N2M0, advanced stage nasopharyngeal cancer.

2 Evidence-Based Treatment Approaches

Radiotherapy (RT) alone is the standard treatment for stage I (Category IB). Concurrent chemoradiotherapy (CRT) is the current standard of care for non-metastatic advanced stage (stages III, IVA, and IVB) nasopharyngeal carcinoma, with or without induction or adjuvant chemotherapy (Category IA). For

Fig. 6.2 MRI coronal image displays minimally extending intracranially through foramen ovale

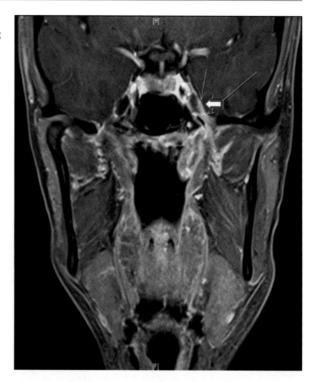

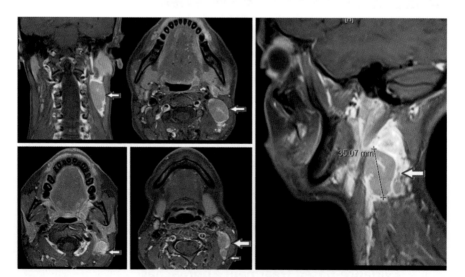

Fig. 6.3 MRI images display bilateral nodal disease, largest on left level 2 measuring 3.5 cm

intermediate-risk disease, stage II, it is recommended to give CRT instead of RT alone (Category 2B).

The MDACC series initially clarified the efficacy of RT alone for T1 category, while RT alone was capable of 5-year local control rates of 93, 79, 68, and 53 % for T1, T2, T3, and T4, respectively. Sanguinetti at al pointed out that advanced T category, squamous histology, and cranial nerve deficits were poor prognostic factors for local control [1].

The major data for combined CRT approach is derived from phase III trial of 230 stage II (T1–2N1M0 or T2N0M0 disease with parapharyngeal space involvement; 13 % is stage III based on AJCC 2010 TNM) nasopharyngeal cancer patients randomized into RT plus concurrent weekly cisplatin (30 mg/m^2) versus RT alone [2]. The addition of concurrent cisplatin significantly improved overall survival from 85.8 % for RT alone to 94.5 % for CRT at 5 years; based on improvement in distant metastasis free survival (94.8 % vs. 83.9 %) without any difference in locoregional relapse-free survival (93.0 % vs. 91.1 %).

Addition of chemotherapy to definitive RT increases overall survival by 4–6 % at 5 years while decreases the risk of event by 10 % and the risk of death by 18 %. CRT demonstrated the most pronounced benefit in comparison to induction chemotherapy or adjuvant chemotherapy [3].

Intergroup 0099 (RTOG 8817) trial established a benefit from concurrent (cisplatin 100 mg/m^2 on days 1, 22, and 43) and adjuvant (cisplatin 80 mg/m^2 on day 1 and fluorouracil 1,000 mg/m^2/day, days 1–4, every 4 weeks for three cycles) chemoradiotherapy (70 Gy, 35–39 fractions, 1.8–2.0 Gy/fraction/day) for stage III and IV nasopharyngeal cancer in comparison to RT alone (CRT vs. RT at 3 year, progression-free survival: 69 % vs. 24 %, overall survival: 78 % vs. 47 %; at 5 years in Table 6.1) [4]. Five-year OS and DFS favored CRT arms over RT alone in other Singapore [5], Taiwan [6], Hong Kong [7, 8], and China [9] randomized trials (Table 6.1).

Induction chemotherapy followed by RT alone approach has failed to show an overall survival benefit compared to RT alone (Table 6.2), but induction chemotherapy in addition to RT slightly improved relapse-free and disease-specific survival [17]. However, sequential therapy of induction chemotherapy followed by concurrent chemoradiotherapy started to be a popular alternative to concurrent chemoradiotherapy with adjuvant chemotherapy [18]. A recent phase II randomized trial comparing induction chemotherapy with docetaxel and cisplatin followed by weekly cisplatin concomitant with RT to weekly cisplatin concomitant with RT. Aside from similar quality of life scores, a trend toward improved 3-year progression-free survival with sequential therapy (88 % vs. 60 %, $p = 0.12$) and significant increase in overall survival with sequential therapy (94 % vs. 68 %) were evident [15].

Until results of phase III trials comparing sequential regimens with concurrent chemoradiotherapy alone (GORTEC-NPC2006, Sun Yat-sen University NCT01245959, Singapore NCT00997906, Taiwan NCT00201396, Hong Kong NCT00379262), sequential therapy should still be considered experimental except clinical presentations with high risk of distant metastasis or difficulty to deliver efficient and safe RT such as large primary tumors (T4), high nodal disease burden,

Table 6.1 Prospective randomized trials of concurrent chemoradiotherapy for locally advanced nasopharyngeal cases

Trials	n	Standard arm (RT)	Randomization arm (CRT)	RT	CRT	p	C	CRT	p
				Disease-free survival	Disease-free survival		Overall survival	Overall survival	
Intergroup 0099 [4, 10]	150	70 Gy	70 Gy with cisplatin+3 cycles of cisplatin/5FU	29 %	58 %	<0.001	37 %	67 %	0.005
Singapore trial [5]	221	70 Gy	70 Gy with cisplatin+3 cycles of cisplatin/5FU	53 % (3 years)	72 % (3 years)	0.01	65 %	80 % (3 years)	0.01
Taiwan trial [6]	284	70–74 Gy	70–74 Gy with cisplatin	53 %	72 %	0.0012	(3 years)	72 %	0.0022
Hong Kong trial [7]	348	66 Gy	66 Gy with cisplatin+3 cycles of cisplatin/5FU	62 %	72 %	0.027	54 %	78 %	0.97
China trial [9]	115	70–74 Gy+10 Gy Boost	70–74 Gy+10 Gy Boost with oxaliplatin	83 % (2 years)	96 % (2 years)	0.02	77 %	100 %	0.01
Hong Kong trial [8]	350	66 Gy+10–20 Gy boost	66 Gy+10–20 Gy boost with cisplatin	52 %	60 %	NS	78 %	70 %	0.065
China trial [11]	506	60–66 Gy with cisplatin	60–66 Gy with cisplatin+3 cycles of cisplatin/5FU	84 % (2 years)	86 % (2 years)	0.13	NA	NA	NS

NS not significant, *CRT* chemoradiotherapy, *RT* radiotherapy

Table 6.2 Prospective randomized trials of neoadjuvant chemotherapy for locally advanced nasopharyngeal cases

Trials	n	Standard arm (RT)	Randomization arm (C→RT)	Disease-free survival			Overall survival		
				RT	C→RT	p	C	C→RT	p
International nasopharyngeal cancer study [12]	339	70 Gy	3 cycles of cisplatin+epirubicin+bleomycin and then 70 Gy	40 % (2 years)	54 % (2 years)	<0.001	NA	NA	NS
China study [13]	456	70 Gy	2–3 cycles of cisplatin+bleomycin+5FU and then 70 Gy	49 %	59 %	0.05	56 %	63 %	0.11
AOCOA [14]	334	70 Gy	2–3 cycles of cisplatin+epirubicin and then 70 Gy	42 % (3 years)	48 % (3 years)	NS	71 % (3 years)	78 % (3 years)	NS
Hong Kong trial [15]	65	70 Gy with cisplatin	2 cycles of docetaxel+cisplatin and then 70 Gy with cisplatin	88.2 % (3 years)	59.5 % (3 years)	0.12	67.7 % (3 years)	94.1 % (3 years)	0.012
China trial [16]	338	70 Gy with cisplatin/5FU +4 cycles of cisplatin/5FU	2 cycles of cisplatin/5FU, then 70 Gy with cisplatin/5FU +4 cycles of cisplatin/5FU	78.5 %	82.5 %	0.16	95.9 % (3 years)	94.5 % (3 years)	0.54

NS Not significant, *CRT* chemoradiotherapy, *RT* radiotherapy, *AOCOA* Asian-Oceanian Clinical Oncology Association

supraclavicular disease, and tumor touching the critical structures such as brainstem, optic pathway, or temporal lobes.

3 Target Volume Determination and Delineation Guidelines

3.1 Gross Tumor Volume (GTV)

GTV should include the gross disease at the primary disease site or any grossly involved lymph nodes (>1 cm or nodes with a necrotic center or PET positive) which are determined from CT, MRI, PET-CT, clinical information, and endoscopic findings. The GTV can be subdivided as the primary site (GTVp) and involved gross lymph nodes (GTVn). A thorough contouring required for GTVp based on the exact spreading pattern which can be questioned by tips as follows:

- Anteriorly:
  Is nasal fossa or pterygopalatine fossa (through sphenopalatine foramen) involved?
  Does the tumor extend to foramen rotundum which is a gateway to intracranial fossa?
  Is the inferior orbital fissure intact (extension into the orbital apex and intracranially through the superior orbital fissure)?
- Laterally:
  Is the parapharyngeal space intact (effacement of the fat)?
  Is the medial or lateral pterygoid muscles infiltrated (trismus clinically)?
  Is the retrostyloid compartment intact (the carotid space to cranial nerves IX, X, XI, and XII)?
  Is the jugular foramen intact (gateway to posterior cranial fossa and IX, X, and XI cranial nerves at risk)?
- Posteriorly:
  Are the prevertebral muscles intact?
- Inferiorly:
  Is there extension through submucosal plane into the oropharynx?
- Superiorly:
  Is skull base eroded?
  Is the foramen lacerum intact (VI nerve at risk)?
  Is the foramen ovale intact?
  Is the mandibular nerve in the parapharyngeal space intact (check extension to gasserian ganglion)?
  Is the cavernous sinus infiltrated (III, IV, ophthalmic division of V, and VI nerves at risk)?

3.2 Clinical Target Volume (CTV)

There needs to be 3 CTV volumes based on risk definitions: CTV2, high risk for subclinical disease including microscopic disease and potential routes of spread for primary and nodal tumor, and CTV3, the lower risk subclinical disease such as low anterior neck:

- *CTV1*, covering GTVp and GTVn with a margin of ≥ 5 mm (as low as 1 mm in close proximity to critical structures: chiasm, brain stem, etc.) given circumferentially around the GTV.
- *CTV2* includes the entire nasopharynx, anterior half of the clivus (entire clivus, if involved), skull base (should include foramen ovale and rotundum bilaterally), pterygoid fossa, bilateral upper deep jugular and parapharyngeal space, inferior sphenoid sinus (entire sphenoid sinus if T3–T4), and posterior third of the nasal cavity and maxillary sinuses (to ensure pterygopalatine fossa coverage). The cavernous sinus should be included in high-risk patients (T3, T4, bulky disease involving the roof of the nasopharynx). CTV2 for nodal target is bilateral if both sides of the neck are involved, and it is ipsilateral if contralateral neck does not have any grossly involved lymph node.

Level definition tips to remember the levels are as follows: Submandibular gland and jugular vein interface separates levels IB (submandibular) and IIa; level II (subdigastric-jugulodigastric) follows the jugular vein to the fossa; hyoid and cricoid define the borders of levels II, III (midjugular), and IV (low jugular and supraclavicular); and posterior edge of sternocleidomastoid defines level V (posterior cervical).

If bilateral neck is heavily involved, CTV2 should cover bilateral retropharyngeal, levels Ib (if isolated retropharyngeal nodes or isolated level IV nodes defining low risk for level IB involvement), II, III, IV, and V; however, if lower neck is uninvolved, then CTV2 does not need to cover levels IV and Vb which is treated in elective CTV3.

If ipsilateral neck is involved alone, then CTV2 covers the bilateral retropharyngeal, ipsilateral levels Ib (limited to the anterior border of submandibular gland in low-risk node-positive patients), II, III, IV, and V, and CTV3 covers the contralateral level Ib (avoid if no extensive involvement of the hard palate, nasal cavity, or maxillary antrum), II, III, IV, and V.

If there is no nodal disease (N0 neck), then omit level Ib in the CTV2 and CTV3 (level IV and supraclavicular nodes) bilaterally [19].

3.3 Planning Target Volume (PTV)

PTV is an extra margin around the CTVs to compensate for the variability and uncertainties of treatment setup and internal organ motion. If the institution has not performed a study to define the appropriate magnitude of PTV, a minimum of 5 mm in all directions is used to define each PTV.

3.4 Case Contouring (Fig. 6.4)

- Check coverage of sphenoid sinus.
- Check coverage of the posterior third of the maxillary sinus.

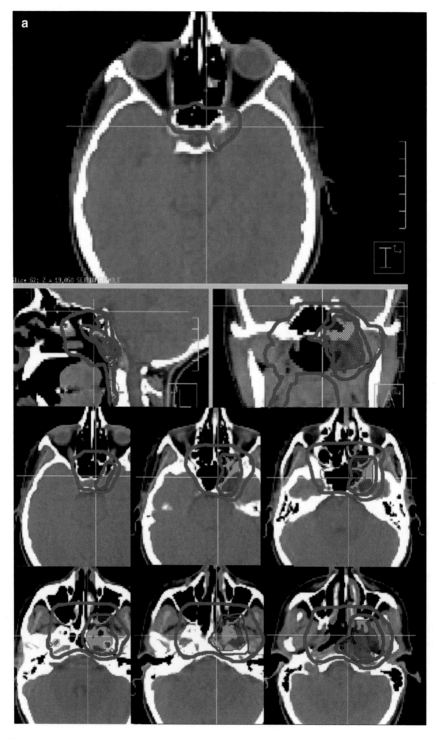

Fig. 6.4 (**a**, **b**) Contouring the CTV1 (*red*), CTV2 (*blue*), and CTV3 (*yellow*)

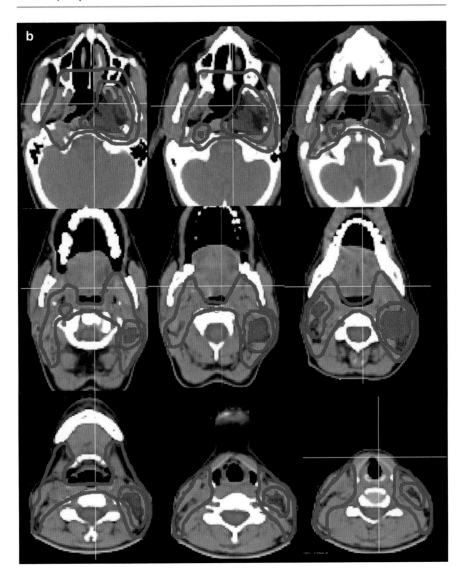

Fig. 6.4 (continued)

- Check coverage of foramen rotundum.
- Check coverage of foramen ovale.
- Check coverage of the half of the clivus and the petroclival fissure.
- Check coverage of ptergopalatine fossa.
- Check coverage of the retrostyloid space.
- Check coverage of soft palate.
- Check coverage of parapharyngeal fat.

4   Treatment Planning

The recommended target volume doses and normal tissue constraints are detailed in
Tables 6.3 and 6.4 (Figs. 6.5, 6.6, 6.7, and 6.8).

- *Treatment Planning Assessment*
  - *Step 1*: Check whether the targets are adequately covered: All plans should be
    normalized to at least 95 % of the volume of PTV70 which is covered by the
    70 Gy isodose surface and 99 % of PTV70 which needs to be at or above
    65.1 Gy. It is confusing to evaluate all PTV DVHs, and one may end up slight
    underdosing of PTV2 and PTV3 when a uniform 3 mm margin is added,
    which is generally 80 % coverage of PTV2 and PTV3 mostly due to parotid
    or a critical structure sparing. However, if your nodal CTVs are relatively
    generous including some muscle outside of the nodal fat plane, much of the
    setup error is "built in" to the CTV contour drawn, so some physicians only
    evaluate CTV2 and CTV3 by looking at dose distributions on the treatment
    plan and not PTV DVH (Fig. 6.8). It is very important to evaluate the DVH of
    PTV1, because a very tight margin on CTV1 could result in underdosing of
    gross disease due to daily setup error. Be careful to ensure that PTV1 should
    receive at least >90 % of prescribed dose.
  - *Step 2*: Check whether there is a large hot spot: No more than 20 % of
    PTV70 is at or above 77Gy and no more than 5 % of PTV70 is at or above
    80 Gy.

Table 6.3 Guidelines for target volume doses

TNM	CTV1 (70Gy/33fr)	CTV2 (59.4–63Gy/33fr)	CTV3 (54–57Gy/33fr)
T1-2 N0	GTVp +1–5 mm	NA	Bilateral RP, Ipsilateral Ib, Bilateral II, III, Va (lower neck – level IV and supraclavicular nodes can be omitted) [19]
T1-4 N1	GTVp+GTVn + 5 mm (1 mm[a])	Ipsilateral Ib–V, Bilateral RP	Contralateral Ib, II–V
T1-4 N2	GTVp+GTVn + 5 mm (1 mm[a])	Ib–V, Bilateral RPLN	Bilateral 4 and 5b if lower neck is uninvolved
T1-4 N3	GTVp+GTVn + 5 mm (1 mm[a])	Ib–V, Bilateral RPLN	NA

[a]Margin next to critical organs as brain stem, optic pathway structures

Table 6.4 Guidelines for target volume doses guidelines for normal tissue constraints

Structure	Constraints
Brain	<50 Gy
	<30 Gy for large volumes
Brainstem	<54 Gy (no more than 1 % to exceed 60 Gy)
Spinal cord (Fig. 6.5)	<45 Gy (no more than 1 % to exceed 50 Gy)
Optic nerves (Fig. 6.7)	<50 Gy (54 Gy max dose)
Chiasm (Fig. 6.7)	<50 Gy (54 Gy max dose)
Mandible (TM joint)	<69 Gy (No more than 1 cc to exceed 75 Gy)
Brachial plexus	<66 Gy
Oral cavity (excluding PTVs)	Mean dose<40 Gy
Submandibular/sublingual glands	As low as possible
Parotid glands	Mean dose<26 Gy
(Fig. 6.6)	At least 20 cc of the combined volume of both parotid glands<20 Gy
	At least 50 % of one gland<30 Gy (in at least one gland).
Esophagus, postcricoid pharynx (Fig. 6.5)	Mean dose<45 Gy
Each cochlea (Fig. 6.5)	No more than 5 % receives 55 Gy or more
Eyes (Fig. 6.7)	Max dose<50 Gy
Lens (Fig. 6.7)	Max dose<10 Gy, try to achieve<5Gy (as low as possible)
Glottic larynx (Fig. 6.5)	Mean dose<36–45 Gy

- – *Step 3*: Check whether the normal tissue constraints are met.
- – *Step 4*: Check whether the hot/cold spots exist in the wrong place (slide by slide by looking at isodose distribution): The hot spots needs to be arranged in the GTV, and it is necessary to make sure that the hot spot is not on a nerve in the CTV.
- • *Case plan* for above T4N2M0 nasopharyngeal cancer (Fig. 6.9)
  - – Check the dose coverage in sagittal, axial, and coronal images to ensure that all hotspots are in GTV or in CTV70.
  - – Check all axial slides to ensure that all CTVs are adequately covered.
  - – Check the entire nasopharynx, anterior half of the clivus, skull base including foramen ovale and rotundum bilaterally, pterygoid fossa, bilateral upper deep jugular and parapharyngeal space, entire sphenoid sinus and posterior third of the nasal cavity, and posterior maxillary sinuses to ensure pterygopalatine fossa coverage.
  - – Check the well separation of 57 and 63 Gy lines on bilateral neck at the level of larynx, esophagus, and postcricoid pharynx.
  - – Check that no hot spots remain in larynx.

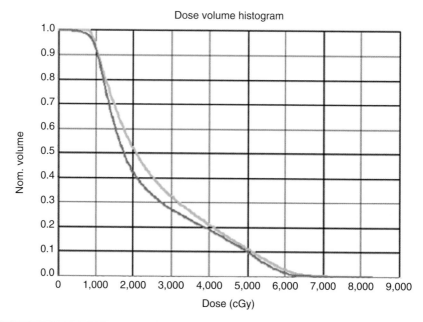

Line Type	ROI	Trial	Min.	Max.	Mean	Std.Dev.
◇ ▬	l parotis	Treatment	376.6	7,116.1	2,606.6	1,521.3
◇ ▬	r parotis	Treatment	--	6,665.0	2,380.8	1,484.6

Fig. 6.5 Dose volume histogram of cochleas, cord, esophagus, and larynx

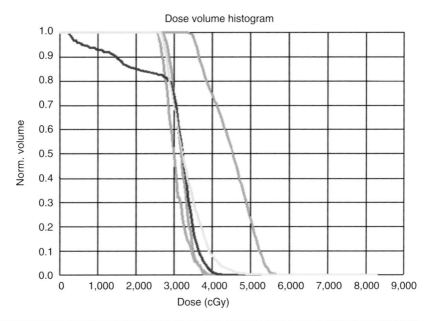

Line type	ROI	Trial	Min.	Max.	Mean	Std.Dev.
	L cochlea	Treatment	2,534.3	3,869.0	3,026.4	285.2
	R cochlea	Treatment	2,675.4	3,774.3	3,181.6	236.5
	Cord	Treatment	232.3	4,238.2	2,695.0	1,188.0
	esophagus	Treatment	3,243.4	5,680.5	4,477.1	579.5
	larynk	Treatment	2,642.9	5,284.2	3,304.8	448.2

Fig. 6.6 Dose volume histogram of parotid glands

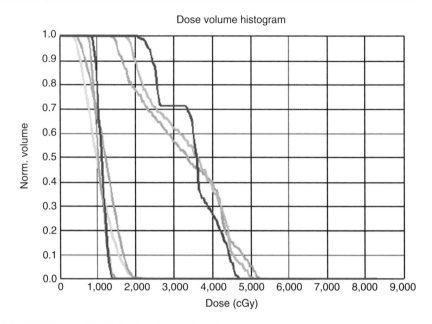

Line type	ROI	Trial	Min.	Max.	Mean	Std.Dev.
	Eye_L	Treatment	347.8	2,098.5	1,017.1	379.0
	Eye_R	Treatment	448.5	2,152.5	1,196.5	366.2
	L optic nerve	Treatment	1,379.1	5,190.6	3,260.1	1,168.5
	Lens_L	Treatment	754.0	1,454.8	1,050.5	169.0
	Lens_R	Treatment	869.8	1,370.1	1,113.7	120.7
	R optic nerve	Treatment	1,754.1	5,021.0	3,388.8	995.1
	chiasm	Treatment	2,060.1	4,676.0	3,473.8	721.4

Fig. 6.7 Dose volume histogram of eyes, optic nerves, and chiasm

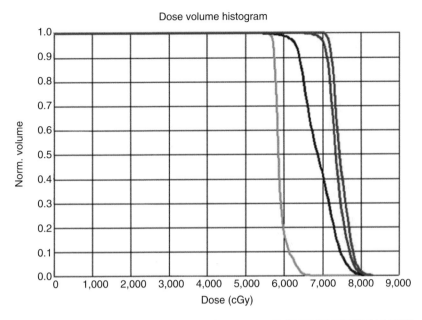

Line type	ROI	Trial	Min.	Max.	Mean	Std.Dev.
ROI statistics						
◇ ━━	CTV57	Treatment	5,230.8	6,651.0	5,900.5	161.9
◇ ━━	CTV63	Treatment	3,608.6	8,271.0	6,891.0	432.1
◇ ━━	CTV70	Treatment	5,062.4	8,271.0	7,370.2	236.9
◇ ━━	GTV	Treatment	6,876.9	8,271.0	7,480.4	213.1

Fig. 6.8 Dose volume histogram of target CTVs: CTV1, CTV2, CTV3

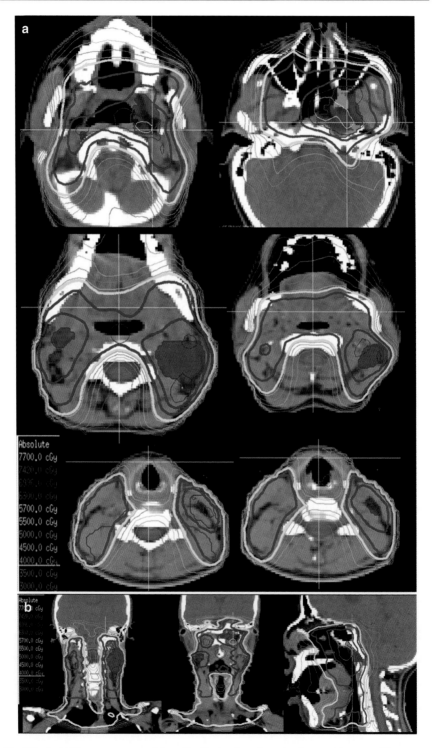

Fig. 6.9 (**a, b**) Dose coverage and dose distribution based on simultaneous integrated boost prescription of 70 Gy to CTV1 (*red*), 63 Gy to CTV2 (*blue*), and 57 Gy to CTV3 (*yellow*)

4.1   Treatment Algorithm and Follow-up

Recommended algorithms for the treatment and follow up of nasopharyngeal cancers are summarized in Figures 6.10 and 6.11.

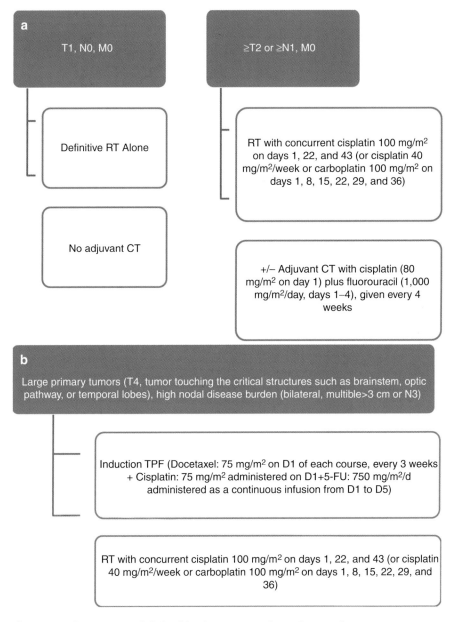

Fig. 6.10 (**a**, **b**) Recommended algorithm for treatment of nasopharyngeal cancer

Fig. 6.11 Recommended algorithm for follow-up of nasopharyngeal cancer

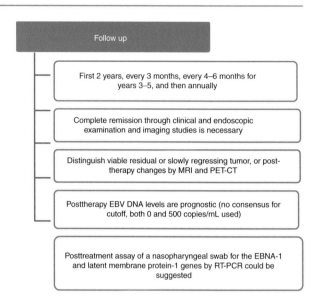

Follow up

First 2 years, every 3 months, every 4–6 months for years 3–5, and then annually

Complete remission through clinical and endoscopic examination and imaging studies is necessary

Distinguish viable residual or slowly regressing tumor, or post-therapy changes by MRI and PET-CT

Posttherapy EBV DNA levels are prognostic (no consensus for cutoff, both 0 and 500 copies/mL used)

Posttreatment assay of a nasopharyngeal swab for the EBNA-1 and latent membrane protein-1 genes by RT-PCR could be suggested

References

1. Sanguineti G, Geara FB, Garden AS, Tucker SL, Ang KK, Morrison WH, Peters LJ (1997) Carcinoma of the nasopharynx treated by radiotherapy alone: determinants of local and regional control. Int J Radiat Oncol Biol Phys 37(5):985–996
2. Chen QY, Wen YF, Guo L, Liu H, Huang PY, Mo HY, Li NW, Xiang YQ, Luo DH, Qiu F et al (2011) Concurrent chemoradiotherapy vs radiotherapy alone in stage II nasopharyngeal carcinoma: phase III randomized trial. J Natl Cancer Inst 103(23):1761–1770
3. Baujat B, Audry H, Bourhis J, Chan AT, Onat H, Chua DT, Kwong DL, Al-Sarraf M, Chi KH, Hareyama M et al (2006) Chemotherapy in locally advanced nasopharyngeal carcinoma: an individual patient data meta-analysis of eight randomized trials and 1753 patients. Int J Radiat Oncol Biol Phys 64(1):47–56
4. Al-Sarraf M, LeBlanc M, Giri PG, Fu KK, Cooper J, Vuong T, Forastiere AA, Adams G, Sakr WA, Schuller DE et al (1998) Chemoradiotherapy versus radiotherapy in patients with advanced nasopharyngeal cancer: phase III randomized Intergroup study 0099. J Clin Oncol 16(4):1310–1317
5. Wee J, Tan EH, Tai BC, Wong HB, Leong SS, Tan T, Chua ET, Yang E, Lee KM, Fong KW et al (2005) Randomized trial of radiotherapy versus concurrent chemoradiotherapy followed by adjuvant chemotherapy in patients with American Joint Committee on Cancer/International Union against cancer stage III and IV nasopharyngeal cancer of the endemic variety. J Clin Oncol 23(27):6730–6738
6. Lin JC, Jan JS, Hsu CY, Liang WM, Jiang RS, Wang WY (2003) Phase III study of concurrent chemoradiotherapy versus radiotherapy alone for advanced nasopharyngeal carcinoma: positive effect on overall and progression-free survival. J Clin Oncol 21(4):631–637
7. Lee AW, Tung SY, Chua DT, Ngan RK, Chappell R, Tung R, Siu L, Ng WT, Sze WK, Au GK et al (2010) Randomized trial of radiotherapy plus concurrent-adjuvant chemotherapy vs radiotherapy alone for regionally advanced nasopharyngeal carcinoma. J Natl Cancer Inst 102(15):1188–1198
8. Chan AT, Leung SF, Ngan RK, Teo PM, Lau WH, Kwan WH, Hui EP, Yiu HY, Yeo W, Cheung FY et al (2005) Overall survival after concurrent cisplatin-radiotherapy compared with

radiotherapy alone in locoregionally advanced nasopharyngeal carcinoma. J Natl Cancer Inst 97(7):536–539

9. Zhang L, Zhao C, Peng PJ, Lu LX, Huang PY, Han F, Wu SX (2005) Phase III study comparing standard radiotherapy with or without weekly oxaliplatin in treatment of locoregionally advanced nasopharyngeal carcinoma: preliminary results. J Clin Oncol 23(33):8461–8468

10. Al-Sarraf M, LeBlanc M, Giri PG, Fu KK, Cooper J, Vuong T, Forastiere AA, Adams G, Sakr WA, Schuller DE et al (2001) Superiority of 5-year survival with chemoradiotherapy vs. radiotherapy in patients with locally advanced nasopharyngeal cancer. Intergroup 0099 Phase III Study. Final report. Proc Am Soc Clin Oncol 20:2279

11. Chen L, Hu CS, Chen XZ, Hu GQ, Cheng ZB, Sun Y, Li WX, Chen YY, Xie FY, Liang SB et al (2012) Concurrent chemoradiotherapy plus adjuvant chemotherapy versus concurrent chemoradiotherapy alone in patients with locoregionally advanced nasopharyngeal carcinoma: a phase 3 multicentre randomised controlled trial. Lancet Oncol 13(2):163–171

12. International Nasopharynx Cancer Study Group, VUMCA I Trial (1996) Preliminary results of a randomized trial comparing neoadjuvant chemotherapy (cisplatin, epirubicin, bleomycin) plus radiotherapy vs. radiotherapy alone in stage IV(>or=N2, M0) undifferentiated nasopharyngeal carcinoma: a positive effect on progression-free survival. Int J Radiat Oncol Biol Phys 35(3):463–469

13. Ma J, Mai HQ, Hong MH, Min HQ, Mao ZD, Cui NJ, Lu TX, Mo HY (2001) Results of a prospective randomized trial comparing neoadjuvant chemotherapy plus radiotherapy with radiotherapy alone in patients with locoregionally advanced nasopharyngeal carcinoma. J Clin Oncol 19(5):1350–1357

14. Chua DT, Sham JS, Choy D, Lorvidhaya V, Sumitsawan Y, Thongprasert S, Vootiprux V, Cheirsilpa A, Azhar T, Reksodiputro AH (1998) Preliminary report of the Asian-Oceanian Clinical Oncology Association randomized trial comparing cisplatin and epirubicin followed by radiotherapy versus radiotherapy alone in the treatment of patients with locoregionally advanced nasopharyngeal carcinoma. Asian-Oceanian Clinical Oncology Association Nasopharynx Cancer Study Group. Cancer 83(11):2270–2283

15. Hui EP, Ma BB, Leung SF, King AD, Mo F, Kam MK, Yu BK, Chiu SK, Kwan WH, Ho R et al (2009) Randomized phase II trial of concurrent cisplatin-radiotherapy with or without neoadjuvant docetaxel and cisplatin in advanced nasopharyngeal carcinoma. J Clin Oncol 27(2):242–249

16. Xu T, Hu C, Zhu G, He X, Wu Y, Ying H (2012) Preliminary results of a phase III randomized study comparing chemotherapy neoadjuvantly or concurrently with radiotherapy for locoregionally advanced nasopharyngeal carcinoma. Med Oncol 29(1):272–278

17. Langendijk JA, Leemans CR, Buter J, Berkhof J, Slotman BJ (2004) The additional value of chemotherapy to radiotherapy in locally advanced nasopharyngeal carcinoma: a meta-analysis of the published literature. J Clin Oncol 22(22):4604–4612

18. OuYang PY, Xie C, Mao YP, Zhang Y, Liang XX, Su Z, Liu Q, Xie FY (2013) Significant efficacies of neoadjuvant and adjuvant chemotherapy for nasopharyngeal carcinoma by meta-analysis of published literature-based randomized, controlled trials. Ann Oncol 24(8):2136–2146

19. Li JG, Yuan X, Zhang LL, Tang YQ, Liu L, Chen XD, Gong XC, Wan GF, Liao YL, Ye JM et al (2013) A randomized clinical trial comparing prophylactic upper versus whole-neck irradiation in the treatment of patients with node-negative nasopharyngeal carcinoma. Cancer 119(17):3170–3176

Oropharynx

7

Ugur Selek, Yasemin Bolukbasi, Yucel Saglam,
Erkan Topkan, and Gokhan Ozyigit

> **Overview**
>
> *Epidemiology*
>
> Historically tobacco and alcohol use were the major risk factors, though human papillomavirus (HPV) infection related increase in incidence is a current fact particularly in younger adults.
>
> *Pathological and Biological Features*
>
> Squamous cell oropharyngeal cancer can be well-, moderately, or poorly differentiated. As HPV relation might propose better prognosis, no evidence exists to indicate treatment is different from other types.
>
> *Definitive Therapy*
>
> Single modality radiotherapy or primary surgery for early-stage disease, individually decided based on related morbidity, has retrospectively generated similar rates of local control and survival, as no prospective randomized

U. Selek, MD (✉)
Department of Radiation Oncology, Koc University, Faculty of Medicine, Istanbul, Turkey

Department of Radiation Oncology, University of Texas MD Anderson Cancer Center, Houston, TX, USA
e-mail: ugurselek@yahoo.com

Y. Bolukbasi, MD • Y. Saglam, MSc
Department of Radiation Oncology, MD Anderson Radiation Treatment Center, American Hospital, Nisantasi, Istanbul, Turkey

E. Topkan, MD
Department of Radiation Oncology, Baskent University, Faculty of Medicine, Adana, Turkey

G. Ozyigit, MD
Department of Radiation Oncology, Hacettepe University, Faculty of Medicine, Sihhiye, Ankara, Turkey

© Springer International Publishing Switzerland 2015
M. Beyzadeoglu et al. (eds.), *Radiation Therapy for Head and Neck Cancers: A Case-Based Review*, DOI 10.1007/978-3-319-10413-3_7

comparison is present. Except for well-lateralized tonsil primaries, bilateral neck requires elective treatment.

Locally advanced stages III and IVA/B cancers without distant metastases require a multidisciplinary approach with more than one modality. Modern surgical approaches with functional preservation for patients with potentially resectable, locally advanced cancer are increasing in frequency as an acceptable initial option, followed by radiation therapy (RT) or chemoradiotherapy. Functional organ preservation approaches with concurrent chemotherapy and RT without surgery is most preferred alternative.

Adjuvant Therapy
Postoperative RT with or without concurrent chemotherapy is recommended for those with high-risk features (positive or close resection margins, nodal extracapsular extension, lymphovascular and perineural invasion).

1   Case Presentation

Sixty-nine-year-old male who was an ex-smoker with 30 pack-year history of smoking presented with a difficulty in swallowing and pain behind his tongue, an obstruction feeling in his throat, and 2 weeks old left neck swelling, without trismus, odynophagia, otalgia, new voice changes, change in his cough or sputum, hemoptysis, dyspnea, aspiration, or weight loss. He had a significant past medical history with coronary artery disease but has denied any chest pain, palpitations, or shortness of breath.

His physical exam revealed normal external ear canals and tympanic membranes with appropriate light reflex. Nasal septum was midline without deviation and was clear to anterior rhinoscopy. There was a large tumor localized in left tonsillar area extending to left anterior tonsillar pillar and base of tongue which was narrowing the airway, and left base of tongue sounded gross invasion with tumor, while there were no lesions of the gingiva, buccal mucosa, floor of mouth, and oral tongue by visualization or palpation. He had moderate dentition. Palate elevates asymmetrically with the bulk on left side. Tongue protrudes normally. There was an approximately 3 cm hardly mobile node in the left upper level II area and was no other palpable adenopathy contralaterally. Cranial nerves II–XII are grossly intact without any facial numbness. The scope was introduced into the left nasal cavity. Clearly seen was normal nasopharyngeal mucosa and bilateral fossa of Rosenmuller. As the scope was advanced, there was narrowed airway with a left-sided bulk of tumor in left tonsillar area which was extending to left anterior tonsillar pillar, to base of tongue, and inferiorly to left aryepiglottic plica. The scope was advanced further. There was no evidence of disease in the larynx and hypopharynx. Vocal cords were mobile. Both MRI and PET-CT defined an oropharyngeal left palatine tonsillar tumor (5×3.5×3.5 cm) extending superiorly to left anterior tonsillar pillar, anterior inferiorly to base of tongue, inferiorly to left aryepiglottic plica which is narrowing glossopharyngeal recess and oro/hypopharyngeal airway without any sign of pre-vertebral fascial invasion, in addition to two pathologic nodes on left neck level 2 (3.2 cm and 8 mm) (Fig. 7.1a, b). A biopsy was performed from the prominent tumor confirming moderately differentiated squamous cell carcinoma. He was staged as T3N2bM0, advanced stage oropharyngeal cancer.

2 Evidence-Based Treatment Approaches

Single modality radiotherapy or primary surgery (transoral or open resection) for stage T1-2 N0-1 has been preferred with similar rates of local control and survival, as no prospective randomized comparison is present [1–3]. Concurrent chemoradio-therapy is mostly the key treatment for locally advanced stages III and IVA/B cancers without distant metastases (Table 7.1) [4–11], while the resectability and neck nodal disease volume are denominators in decision making to perform initially surgery for primary (T3–T4a) and neck (N0-1) and to consolidate with radiotherapy (close resection margins, lymphovascular and perineural invasion, pT3-T4, N2 or N3, nodal disease levels IV–V) or chemoradiotherapy (positive surgical margins and/or nodal extracapsular invasion) metastases (Table 7.2) [12–15]. Induction chemotherapy fol-lowed by radio/chemoradiotherapy is yet a category three approach which might be considered in heavy nodal volume with an increased risk of distant metastases [5, 6, 16–19]. Cetuximab as a single agent concurrent with radiotherapy for treatment of locoregionally advanced head and neck cancer seemed to improve locoregional con-trol and to reduce mortality, while the addition of cetuximab to the chemoradiother-apy with cisplatin did not improve progression-free or overall survival [20].

It has become evident as one of the most significant recent advances that HPV-positive oropharyngeal cancer (HPVOPC) should be considered as a different entity from HPV-negative cancers [21]. HPVOPC is frequently presenting with a smaller primary tumor and more advanced cervical lymph node disease which is having a cystic appearance [22–24].

Oropharyngeal cancer has been recommended to be classified as having a low (HPV+, ≤10 pack-year smoking or >10 pack-year and N0–N2a), intermediate (HPV+, >10 pack-year smoking and N2b–N3 or HPV-, ≤10 pack-year smoking, T2–3), or high risk (HPV-, ≤10 pack-year smoking, T4 or HPV-, >10 pack-year smoking) of death on the basis of four factors [25, 26]. However, as the results of ongoing trials for metastases (Table 7.3) are incomplete, current recommendation should be treatment regardless of the HPV status according to the stage of disease at presentation.

3 Target Volume Determination and Delineation Guidelines

Oropharynx is shaped with following structures: palatoglossal arch, pharyngeal ton-sil, tonsillar fossa, tonsillar pillar, palatopharyngeal arch, base of the tongue, epi-glottic vallecula, posterior wall of the oropharynx, and oral surface of the soft palate,

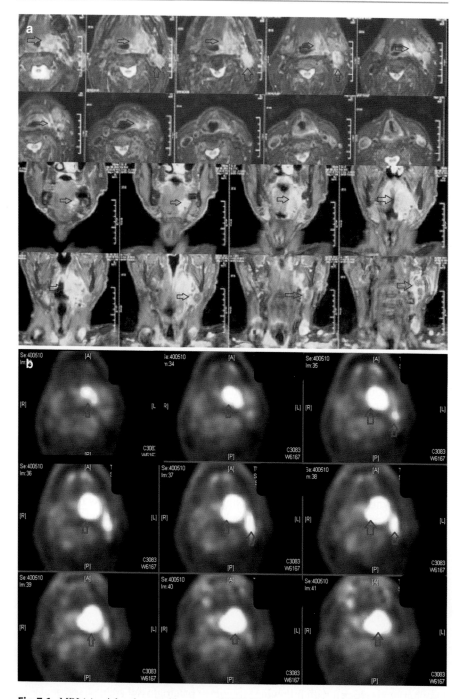

Fig. 7.1 MRI (**a**) axial and coronal images and PET-CT (**b**) display an oropharyngeal left palatine tonsillar tumor extending superiorly to left anterior tonsillar pillar, anterior inferiorly to base of tongue, and inferiorly to left aryepiglottic plica which is narrowing glossopharyngeal recess and oro/hypopharyngeal airway

Table 7.1 Large, randomized phase III trials of concurrent chemoradiation

Trial	Year	N	RT Standard	Schedule Comparison	Concomitant CT	DFS or PFS RT	CRT	OS RT	CRT	Conclusion
French [4] GORTEC 94-01	2004	226	70 Gy; 2 Gy/fraction	70 Gy; 2 Gy/fraction	3 cycles of carboplatin+5FU	14.6	26.6	15.8	22.4	Chemoradiotherapy improved overall survival and locoregional control
Swiss [8] SAKK	2004	224	74.4 Gy; 1.2 Gy/fraction twice daily	74.4 Gy; 1.2 Gy/fraction twice daily	2 cycles of cisplatin	–	–	32	46	Therapeutic index of radiotherapy is enhanced by concurrent cisplatin
German [9] 95-06	2005	384	30 Gy; 2 Gy/fraction+40.6 Gy; 1.4 Gy/fraction twice daily to a total of 70.6 Gy	14 Gy; 2 Gy/fraction+63.6 Gy; 1.4 Gy/fraction twice daily to a total of 77.6 Gy	5FU+mitomycin	26.6	29.3	23.7	28.6	C-HART (70.6 Gy) is superior to dose-escalated HART (77.6 Gy)
FNCLCC/ GORTEC [10]	2006	163	80.4 Gy; 1.2 Gy/fraction twice daily, 5 days per week	80.4 Gy; 1.2 Gy/fraction twice daily, 5 days per week	3 cycles of Cisplatin+5FU	25.2 (2 y)	48.2 (2 y)	20.1 (2 y)	37.8 (2 y)	Chemoradiotherapy reveals better outcome than radiotherapy alone, even with an aggressive dose-intense schedule
RTOG 0129 [11]	2010	743	70 Gy; 2 Gy/fraction	72 Gy; 42 fractions over 6 weeks	2–3 cycles of cisplatin	–	–	59	56	Standard of care for these patients remains concurrent chemoradiotherapy with standard fractionation.

N number of patients, *RT* radiotherapy, *CT* chemotherapy, *OS* overall survival, *DFS* disease-free survival, *PFS* progression-free survival

Table 7.2 Two concurrent postoperative radiation plus chemotherapy trials

Trial		RTOG 9501 [14, 15]	EORTC 22931 [12]
# patients		416	334
Median follow-up, months		45.9 (120)	60
% oropharyngeal cancer		43	30
Radiotherapy alone		60 Gy in 6 weeks	66 Gy in 6.5 weeks
Chemoradiotherapy		60 Gy in 6 weeks plus cisplatin 100 mg/m² on days 1, 22, and 43	66 Gy in 6.5 weeks plus cisplatin 100 mg/m² on days 1, 22, and 43
Inclusion criteria	Positive resection margin	+ (6 % of patients)	+ (13 % of patients)
	Extracapsular extension	+ (49 % of patients)	+ (41 % of patients)
	≥2 nodes involved	+	−
	Perineural involvement	−	+
	Vascular tumor embolism	−	+
	Oral cavity or oropharyngeal tumor with involvement of level IV or V lymph nodes	−	+
Overall survival	Radiotherapy alone	47 % (27 %)	40 %
	Chemoradiotherapy	56 % (29 %)	53 %
Local-regional recurrence	Radiotherapy alone	33 % (28.8 %)	31 %
	Chemoradiotherapy	22 % (22.3 %)	18 %
Disease free survival	Radiotherapy alone	36 % (19.1 %)	36 %
	Chemoradiotherapy	47 % (20.1 %)	47 %
Conclusion [13]		Subgroup of patients with either microscopically involved resection margins and/or extracapsular spread showed improved local-regional control and disease-free survival by concurrent chemoradiotherapy	

Table 7.3 Ongoing phase 3 randomized trials in HPV-positive or HPV-negative oropharyngeal cancer patients

Trial	HPV status	Inclusion criteria	Exclusion criteria	Treatment
EORTC-1219	(−)	Oropharynx/larynx/hypopharynx primary tumor, stage III or IV (M0)	−	Accelerated 70 Gy in 6 weeks RT plus cisplatin vs accelerated
				RT plus cisplatin plus nimorazole
RTOG-1016	(+)	T1–2,N2a–N3 or T3–4,any N	−	Accelerated 70 Gy IMRT plus high-dose cisplatin vs accelerated IMRT plus cetuximab
TROG 12.01	(+)	Stage III (excluding T1–2 N1) or IV if ≤10 pack-year smoking history If >10 pack-year smoking history, only N0–N2a	T4, N3, or M1	RT plus weekly cetuximab vs RT plus weekly cisplatin
The Quarterback Trial	(+)	Oropharynx/unknown primary/nasopharynx, stage III or IV disease (M0),	Active smokers or smoking >20 pack-year	Responders of 3 cycles of induction TPF randomized to 70 Gy RT plus weekly carbo-platin vs RT (56 Gy) plus weekly carboplatin plus cetuximab
De-ESCALaTE	(+)	Stage III–Iva (T3N0–T4N0, and T1N1–T4N3) ≥N2b disease and smoking history	>10 pack-year excluded	RT plus high-dose cisplatin vs RT plus cetuximab
ADEPT	(+)	Transoral resection (R0 margin) T1–4a, pN-positive with extracapsular spread	−	60 Gy IMRT in 6 weeks vs IMRT plus cisplatin

uvula. The most common locations for a primary tumor of the oropharynx are anterior tonsillar pillar and tonsil. Primary lymphatic drainage is the retropharyngeal, level II and III nodes.

Gross Tumor Volume (GTV)

GTV should include the gross disease at the primary disease site or any grossly involved lymph nodes (>1 cm or nodes with a necrotic center or PET positive) which are determined from CT, MRI, PET-CT, clinical information, and endoscopic findings [27]. The GTV can be subdivided as the primary site (GTVp) and involved gross lymph nodes (GTVn). A thorough contouring is required for GTVp based on the exact spreading pattern which can be questioned as follows given two major sites, base of tongue and tonsil:

- Anteriorly:
  Is lingual surface of epiglottis involved (T3 for tonsil primary, T does not change for base of tongue or vallecula primary)?
  Is retromolar trigone involved?
  Is buccal mucosa involved (drainage to buccal nodes)?
  Is anterior tonsillar pillar involved?
  Is tonsillar fossa involved (lymphatic drainage is primarily to level V nodes)?
  Is oral tongue involved (IA drainage, T stage does not change; intrinsic muscles – no bony attachment)?
  Is the mandible involved (T4a)?
- Laterally:
  Is the medial (T4a) or lateral pterygoid (T4b) muscles infiltrated (trismus clinically)?
  Is the retrostyloid compartment intact (the carotid space to cranial nerves IX, X, XI, and XII)?
  Is the jugular foramen intact (gateway to posterior cranial fossa and IX, X, and XI cranial nerves at risk)?
- Posteriorly:
  Is posterior tonsillar pillar involved (possible inferior extension to the pharyngo-epiglottic fold and posterior aspect of the thyroid cartilage; more frequent involvement for level V nodes)?
  Is the prevertebral fascia infiltrated?
- Inferiorly:
  Is the floor of the mouth involved (T4a; extrinsic muscles – with bony attachment as hyo/genio/palato/styloglossus; mylohyoid muscle which separates sublingual and submandibular space)?
  Is the larynx involved?
  Is the pyriform sinus involved?
  Is the hypopharyngeal wall involved?
- Superiorly:
  Is the soft palate involved?
  Is hard palate involved (T4a)?

Clinical Target Volume (CTV)

There needs to be three CTV volumes based on risk definitions while respecting anatomical barriers (air, muscle, skin, bone, etc.) to microscopic spread.

- CTV 1, covering GTVp and GTVn with a margin of ≥ 5 mm (as low as 1 mm in close proximity to critical structures: chiasm, brain stem, etc.) given circumferentially around the GTV.
- CTV 2, high risk for subclinical disease including microscopic disease and potential routes of spread for primary and nodal tumor.
- CTV 3, the lower risk subclinical disease such as low anterior neck.

Tonsil CTV1p

- Contours in air being trimmed after expansion of GTV with 8–10 mm will help planning.
- CTV1 of tonsil primary should be considered a region/territory in contrast to a uniform expansion performed in base of tongue primary.
- Maxillary tuberosity should be covered.
- Ipsilateral base of tongue should be minimally (≈3 mm) covered, even if there is no base of tongue extension of GTV.
- Ipsilateral glossopharyngeal sulcus should be minimally (≈3 mm) covered.
- Ipsilateral retromolar trigone should be covered.
- The lower margin of CTV1p should cover the superior tip of hyoid inferiorly.

Tonsil CTV2

- Ipsilateral soft and hard palate is required to be covered to midline.
- Ipsilateral glossotonsillar sulcus (separation of tonsillar area from the base of the tongue; between anterior tonsillar pillar and pharyngoepiglottic fold) is necessary to be covered anteriorly and inferiorly.
- Ipsilateral base of tongue is covered.
- Pterygoid plate is recommended to be included (in CTV3 if N0) to ensure pterygomandibular raphe (pterygomandibular ligament between medial pterygoid plate and mylohyoid line of mandible) coverage.
- Whole lateral pterygoid muscle needs coverage if there is trismus or radiological involvement, though less than half of muscle is enough to be covered if no extension.
- Ipsilateral lateral pharyngeal wall needs to be covered until at least to aryepiglottic fold inferiorly.
- Ipsilateral parapharyngeal space is covered to secure inclusion of microscopic local extension of primary besides retropharyngeal and parapharyngeal nodal involvement.
- Parotids should be covered as required in case of gross disease bordering.

- Nodal treatment can be limited to ipsilateral neck alone to spare contralateral neck if tonsil primary is small (T1), well lateralized, node negative, or low bulk N1, without extension to soft palate or base of tongue.
- Node-positive site requires levels IB–V coverage in CTV2n, while IB–IV or IB–V is dictated based on location of nodal disease, low neck CTV3 might not involve level V.
- Ipsilateral level IB could be in CTV2 or might be covered in CTV3 if the involved nodes are farther away. Contralateral level IB might be spared if node negative or level II is not involved, which helps decreasing oral cavity dose.
- Level IA needs coverage if there is extension to oral tongue or oral cavity.
- Retropharyngeal nodal coverage (between medial side of longus colli and lateral to styloids) is required to start at jugular foramen if node positive, though is considered enough to start at tip of atlas or transverse process of C1 if node negative. The coverage should encompass inferiorly to bottom of hyoid or bottom of C2.
- Bilateral retrostyloid spaces are involved in CTV2n; however, it might be omitted if node negative.

Base of Tongue CTV1

- Contours in air being trimmed after expansion of GTV with 8–10 mm will help planning.
- CTV1 is a uniform expansion for base of tongue primary in contrast to tonsil primary.
- Entire vallecula should be covered if there is extension to vallecula.

Base of Tongue CTV2

- Parotids should be covered as required in case of gross disease bordering.
- It is not necessary to cover pterygoid plates if tonsil is not involved.
- It is not necessary to cover soft palate if tonsil is not involved.
- Remaining base of tongue is covered for > T1, while approximately circumferential 1 cm of remaining base of tongue is enough for well-lateralized T1 tumors.
- Circumferential 8–10 mm margin aside from base of tongue except next to bone is recommended.
- Ipsilateral glossotonsillar sulcus is necessary to be covered anteriorly and inferiorly.
- Preepiglottic space needs coverage of minimum 1–1.5 cm caudal to GTV.
- Ipsilateral posterior pharyngeal wall needs to be covered with at least 1 cm circumferentially over CTV1.

- Node-positive site requires levels IB–V coverage in CTV2n, while IB–IV or IB–V is dictated based on location of nodal disease, low neck CTV3 might not involve level V.
- Ipsilateral level IB could be in CTV2 or might be covered in CTV3 if the involved nodes are farther away. Contralateral level IB might be spared if node negative or level II is not involved, which helps decreasing oral cavity dose.
- IA needs coverage if there is extension to oral tongue or oral cavity.
- Retropharyngeal nodal coverage (between medial side of longus colli and lateral to styloids) is required to start at jugular foramen if node positive; though it is considered enough to start at tip of atlas or transverse process of C1 if node negative. The coverage should encompass inferiorly to bottom of hyoid or bottom of C2.
- Bilateral retrostyloid spaces are involved in CTV2n; however, it might be omitted if node negative.

Planning Target Volume (PTV)

PTV is extra margin around the CTVs to compensate for the variability and uncertainties of treatment setup and internal organ motion. If the institution has not performed a study to define the appropriate magnitude of PTV, a minimum of 5 mm in all directions is used to define each PTV.

Case Contouring (Fig. 7.2)

- Check ipsilateral pterygoid plates contoured in CTV3 and CTV2.
- Check minimum to half of the lateral pterygoid muscle contoured.
- Check contralateral retropharyngeal contouring start at jugular foramen.
- Check tonsillar primary CTV1 including maxillary tuberosity.
- Check remaining soft palate contoured in CTV2.
- Check bilateral retrostyloid spaces contoured.
- Check glossotonsillar sulcus contoured even if not involved ipsilaterally.
- Check remaining base of tongue contoured in CTV2 due to base of tongue invasion.
- Check parapharyngeal space contoured.
- Check ipsilateral retromolar trigone contoured.
- Check lateral pharyngeal wall contoured until aryepiglottic fold.
- Check ipsilateral superior tip of hyoid included in contouring.
- Check level IB not contoured in N0 contralateral neck.
- Check preepiglottic space contoured due to base of tongue invasion.
- Check retropharyngeal contouring stopped below hyoid.

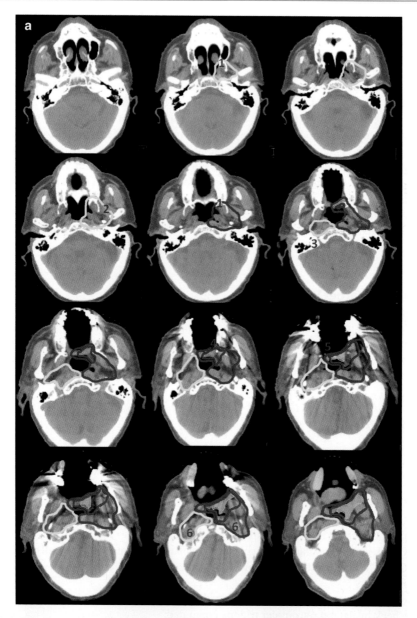

Fig. 7.2 (**a–c**) Contouring the CTV1 (*red*), CTV2 (*blue*), and CTV3 (*yellow*). (**a**)- (*1*) Check ipsilateral pterygoid plates contoured in CTV3 and CTV2, (*2*) check minimum to half of the lateral pterygoid muscle contoured, (*3*) check contralateral retropharyngeal contouring start at jugular foramen, (**b**) (*4*) check tonsillar primary CTV1 including maxillary tuberosity, (*5*) check remaining soft palate contoured in CTV2, (*6*) check bilateral retrostyloid spaces contoured, (**c**) (*7*) check glossotonsillar sulcus contoured even if not involved ipsilaterally, (*8*) check remaining base of tongue contoured in CTV2 due to base of tongue invasion, (*9*) check parapharyngeal space contoured

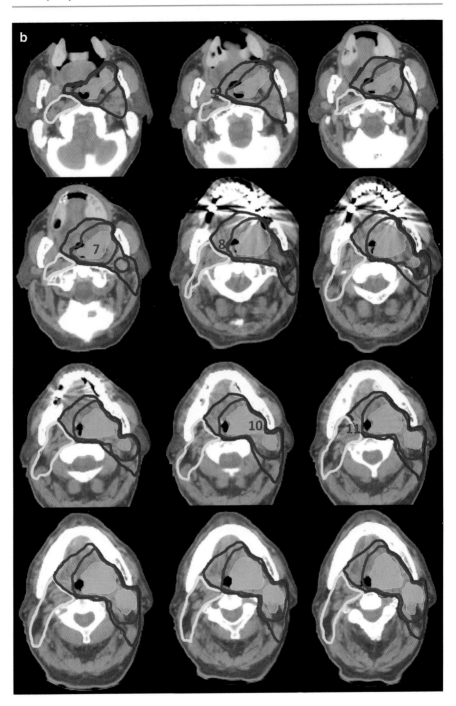

Fig. 7.2 (continued)

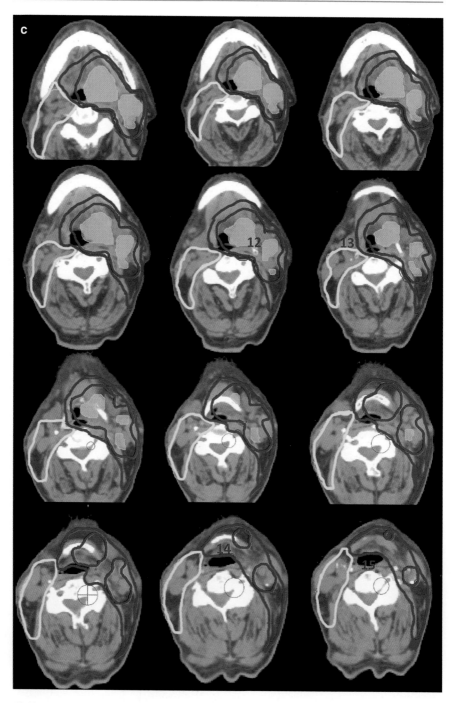

Fig. 7.2 (continued)

Table 7.4 Guidelines for target volume doses for tonsil

TNM	CTV1 (70 Gy/33fr)	CTV2 (59.4–63 Gy/33fr) might be individualized as ≈2 cm below the lowest positive node to continue with CTV for the rest	CTV3 (54–57 Gy/33fr)
N0, small T1 without extension to soft palate or base of tongue, well-lateralized	GTVp +5 mm + tonsillar territory	Ipsilateral Ib, II (Might use CTV3 dose)	Ipsilateral III, IV, and Va (Individualized)
T1–2 N0	GTVp +5 mm + tonsillar territory	Ipsilateral Ib, II–III (Might use CTV3 dose)	Contralateral II–III–IV–Va (individualized) Bilateral RP (Bilateral IV and Vb if lower neck is uninvolved)
T1–4 N1–N2b (single node N3)	GTVp+GTVn	Ipsilateral Ib (Ia if oral tongue involved)	Contralateral II–III–IV–Va
	+ 5 mm + tonsillar territory	Ipsilateral II–III–IV–Va, Ipsilateral RP	Contralateral RP (Bilateral IV and Vb if lower neck is uninvolved)
T1-4N2c-3	GTVp+5 mm+tonsillar territory+GTVn	Bilateral Ib–V RPLN	Bilateral IV and V if lower neck is uninvolved

Tonsillar territory: region including maxillary tuberosity, ipsilateral minimal base of tongue, ipsilateral glossopharyngeal sulcus, ipsilateral retromolar trigone, and superior tip of hyoid

4   Treatment Planning

Guidelines for target volume doses for tonsil carcinoma are summarized in Table 7.4

Guidelines for target volume doses for base of tongue cancers are summarized in Table 7.5.

Guidelines for normal tissue constraints are given in Table 7.6 (Fig. 7.3).

- Treatment Planning Assessment
  - *Step 1*: Check whether the targets are adequately covered. All plans should be normalized to at least 95 % of the volume of PTV70 which is covered by the 70 Gy isodose surface and 99 % of PTV70 which needs to be at or above 65.1 Gy.
  - It is confusing to evaluate all PTV DVHs, and one may end up slight underdosing of PTV2 and PTV3 when a uniform 3 mm margin is added, which is generally 80 % coverage of PTV2 and PTV3 mostly due to parotid or a critical structure sparing.

Table 7.5 Guidelines for target volume doses for base of tongue

TNM	CTV1 (70 Gy/33fr)	CTV2 (59.4–63 Gy/33fr) might be individualized as ≈ 2 cm below the lowest positive node to continue with CTV for the rest	CTV3 (54–57 Gy/33fr)
T1–2 N0	GTVp +5 mm	NA	Bilateral II–III–IV Bilateral RP
T1–4 N1–N2b (single node N3)	GTVp+GTVn + 5 mm	Ipsilateral Ib (Ia if oral tongue involved) Ipsilateral II–III–IV–Va Ipsilateral RP	Contralateral II–III–IV–Va Contralateral RP (Bilateral IV and Vb if lower neck is uninvolved)
T1–4N2c–3	GTVp+GTVn + 5 mm	Ib–Va Bilateral RPLN	Bilateral IV and Vb if lower neck is uninvolved

Table 7.6 Guidelines for normal tissue constraints

Structure	Constraints
Brain	<50 Gy
	<30 Gy for large volumes
Brainstem	<54 Gy (no more than 1 % to exceed 60 Gy)
Spinal cord	<45 Gy (no more than 1 % to exceed 50 Gy)
Optic nerves	<50 Gy (54 Gy max dose)
Chiasm	<50 Gy (54 Gy max dose)
Mandible (TM joint)	<69 Gy (No more than 1 cc to exceed 75 Gy)
Brachial plexus	<66 Gy
Oral cavity (excluding PTVs)	Mean dose<40 Gy
Submandibular/sublingual glands	As low as possible
Parotid glands	Mean dose<26 Gy
	At least 20 cc of the combined volume of both parotid glands <20 Gy
	At least 50 % of one gland<30 Gy (in at least one gland)
Esophagus, postcricoid pharynx	Mean dose<45 Gy
Each cochlea	No more than 5 % receives 55 Gy or more
Eyes	Max dose<50 Gy
Lens	Max dose< 10 Gy, try to achieve<5 Gy (as low as possible)
Glottic larynx	Mean dose<36–45 Gy

– However, if your nodal CTVs are relatively generous including some muscle outside of the nodal fat plane, much of the setup error is "built in" to the CTV contour drawn, so it is mandatory to be decided as a department standard to evaluate CTV2 and CTV3 by looking at dose distributions on the treatment plan and not PTV DVH or to strictly evaluate the PTVs after a tighter contouring for CTVs.

- It is very important to evaluate the DVH of PTV1, because a very tight margin on CTV1 could result in underdosing of gross disease due to daily setup error. Be careful to ensure that PTV1 should receive at least >90 % of prescribed dose.
- *Step 2*: Check whether there is a large hot spot. No more than 20 % of PTV70 is at or above 77 Gy and no more than 5 % of PTV70 is at or above 80 Gy.

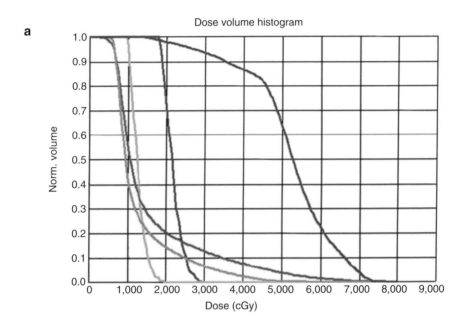

a

Dose volume histogram

ROI Statistics

Line Type	ROI	Trial	Min.	Max.	Mean	Std. Dev.
◇ —	Cochlea, Left	treatment	1772.3	2954.4	2162.6	242.2
◇ —	Cochlea, Right	treatment	954.7	1965.9	1260.2	200.6
◇ —	Parotid , Left	treatment	61.7	7235.1	1553.9	1253.1
◇ —	Parotid , Right	treatment	317.5	5606.8	1261.2	838.3
◇ —	mandibula	treatment	1140.0	7712.1	5170.0	1174.5

Fig. 7.3 (**a**, **b**) Dose volume histogram for organs at risk

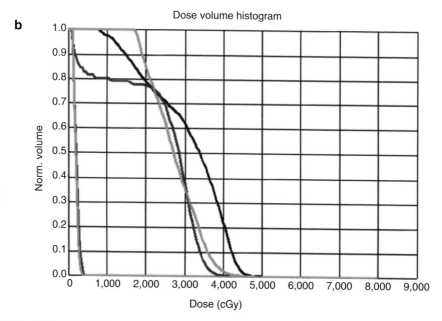

Fig. 7.3 (continued)

- *Step 3*: Check whether the normal tissue constraints are met.
- *Step 4*: Check whether the hot/cold spots exist in the wrong place (slide by slide by looking at isodose distribution). The hot spots need to be arranged in the GTV, and it is necessary to make sure that the hot spot is not on a nerve in the CTV.
- *Case Plan* for Above T3N2bM0 Oropharyngeal Cancer (Fig. 7.4)
- Check the dose coverage in sagittal, axial, and coronal images to ensure that all hot spots are in GTV or in CTV70 (#1).
- Check all axial slides to ensure that all CTVs are adequately covered.

- Check coverage of tonsillar primary CTV1 including maxillary tuberosity (#2), ipsilateral base of tongue (#3), ipsilateral retromolar trigone (#4), ipsilateral glossopharyngeal sulcus (#5), and superior tip of hyoid (#6).
- Check coverage of base of tongue primary CTV1 including entire vallecula if there is extension.

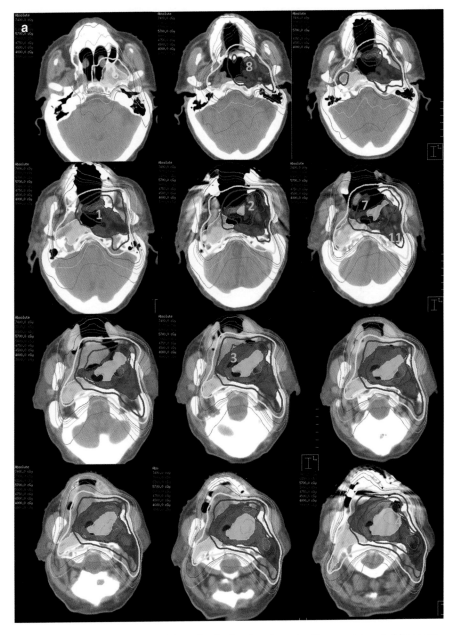

Fig. 7.4 (**a–c**) Dose coverage and dose distribution based on simultaneous integrated boost prescription of 70 Gy to CTV1 (*red*), 63 Gy to CTV2 (*blue*), and 57 Gy to CTV3 (*yellow*)

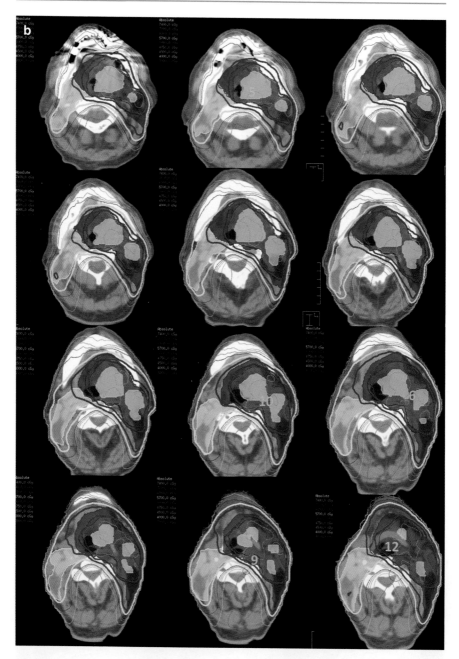

Fig. 7.4 (continued)

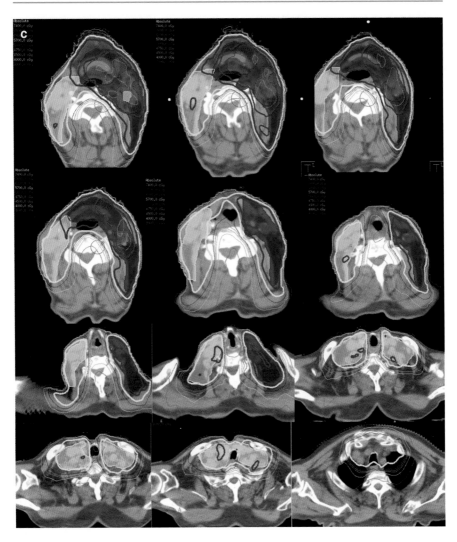

Fig. 7.4 (continued)

– Check coverage of tonsillar primary CTV2 including ipsilateral soft (#7) and hard, ipsilateral glossotonsillar sulcus, ipsilateral base of tongue, ipsilateral pterygoid plate (#8), ipsilateral lateral pterygoid muscle (#8), ipsilateral lateral pharyngeal wall until aryepiglottic fold (#9), ipsilateral parapharyngeal space (#10), retropharyngeal nodes, and bilateral retrostyloid spaces.
– Check coverage of base of tongue primary CTV2 (in this case, major invasion of base of tongue) including remaining base of tongue, ipsilateral glossotonsillar sulcus, preepiglottic space (#12), ipsilateral posterior pharyngeal wall, retropharyngeal nodes, and retrostyloid spaces.
– Check the well separation of 57 and 63 Gy lines on bilateral neck at the level of larynx, esophagus, and postcricoid pharynx.
– Check that no hot spots remain in larynx.

Treatment Algorithm (Fig. 7.5)

Patient Follow-up (Fig. 7.6)

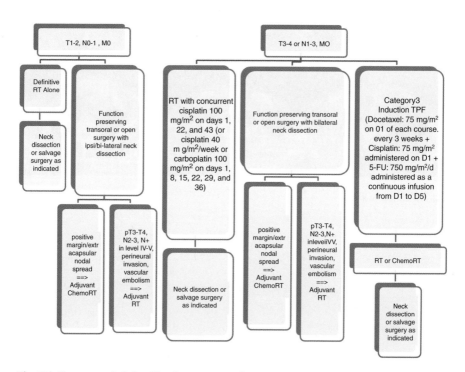

Fig. 7.5 Recommended algorithm for treatment of oropharyngeal cancer

Fig. 7.6 Recommended algorithm for follow-up of oropharyngeal cancer

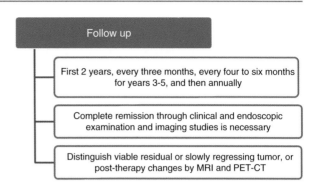

References

1. Adelstein DJ, Ridge JA, Brizel DM, Holsinger FC, Haughey BH, O'Sullivan B, Genden EM, Beitler JJ, Weinstein GS, Quon H et al (2012) Transoral resection of pharyngeal cancer: summary of a National Cancer Institute Head and Neck Cancer Steering Committee Clinical Trials Planning Meeting, November 6–7, 2011, Arlington, Virginia. Head Neck 34(12):1681–1703
2. Li RJ, Richmon JD (2012) Transoral endoscopic surgery: new surgical techniques for oropharyngeal cancer. Otolaryngol Clin North Am 45(4):823–844
3. Selek U, Garden AS, Morrison WH, El-Naggar AK, Rosenthal DI, Ang KK (2004) Radiation therapy for early-stage carcinoma of the oropharynx. Int J Radiat Oncol Biol Phys 59(3):743–751
4. Denis F, Garaud P, Bardet E, Alfonsi M, Sire C, Germain T, Bergerot P, Rhein B, Tortochaux J, Calais G (2004) Final results of the 94–01 French Head and Neck Oncology and Radiotherapy Group randomized trial comparing radiotherapy alone with concomitant radiochemotherapy in advanced-stage oropharynx carcinoma. J Clin Oncol 22(1):69–76
5. Hitt R, Grau JJ, Lopez-Pousa A, Berrocal A, Garcia-Giron C, Irigoyen A, Sastre J, Martinez-Trufero J, Brandariz Castelo JA, Verger E et al (2014) A randomized phase III trial comparing induction chemotherapy followed by chemoradiotherapy versus chemoradiotherapy alone as treatment of unresectable head and neck cancer. Ann Oncol 25(1):216–225
6. Pignon JP, Bourhis J, Domenge C, Designe L (2000) Chemotherapy added to locoregional treatment for head and neck squamous-cell carcinoma: three meta-analyses of updated individual data. MACH-NC Collaborative Group. Meta-Analysis of Chemotherapy on Head and Neck Cancer. Lancet 355(9208):949–955
7. Pignon JP, le Maitre A, Maillard E, Bourhis J (2009) Meta-analysis of chemotherapy in head and neck cancer (MACH-NC): an update on 93 randomised trials and 17,346 patients. Radiother Oncol 92(1):4–14
8. Huguenin P, Beer KT, Allal A, Rufibach K, Friedli C, Davis JB, Pestalozzi B, Schmid S, Thoni A, Ozsahin M et al (2004) Concomitant cisplatin significantly improves locoregional control in advanced head and neck cancers treated with hyperfractionated radiotherapy. J Clin Oncol 22(23):4665–4673
9. Budach V, Stuschke M, Budach W, Baumann M, Geismar D, Grabenbauer G, Lammert I, Jahnke K, Stueben G, Herrmann T et al (2005) Hyperfractionated accelerated chemoradiation with concurrent fluorouracil-mitomycin is more effective than dose-escalated hyperfractionated accelerated radiation therapy alone in locally advanced head and neck cancer: final results of the radiotherapy cooperative clinical trials group of the German Cancer Society 95–06 Prospective Randomized Trial. J Clin Oncol 23(6):1125–1135

10. Bensadoun RJ, Benezery K, Dassonville O, Magne N, Poissonnet G, Ramaioli A, Lemanski C, Bourdin S, Tortochaux J, Peyrade F et al (2006) French multicenter phase III randomized study testing concurrent twice-a-day radiotherapy and cisplatin/5-fluorouracil chemotherapy (BiRCF) in unresectable pharyngeal carcinoma: results at 2 years (FNCLCC-GORTEC). Int J Radiat Oncol Biol Phys 64(4):983–994

11. Ang K, Zhang Q, Wheeler RH, Rosenthal DI, Nguyen-Tan F, Kim H, Lu C, Axelrod RS, Silverman CI, Weber RS (2010) A phase III trial (RTOG 0129) of two radiation-cisplatin regimens for head and neck carcinomas (HNC): impact of radiation and cisplatin intensity on outcome. J Clin Oncol 28(15s):abstr 5507

12. Bernier J, Domenge C, Ozsahin M, Matuszewska K, Lefebvre JL, Greiner RH, Giralt J, Maingon P, Rolland F, Bolla M et al (2004) Postoperative irradiation with or without concomitant chemotherapy for locally advanced head and neck cancer. N Engl J Med 350(19):1945–1952

13. Bernier J, Cooper JS, Pajak TF, van Glabbeke M, Bourhis J, Forastiere A, Ozsahin EM, Jacobs JR, Jassem J, Ang KK et al (2005) Defining risk levels in locally advanced head and neck cancers: a comparative analysis of concurrent postoperative radiation plus chemotherapy trials of the EORTC (#22931) and RTOG (# 9501). Head Neck 27(10):843–850

14. Cooper JS, Pajak TF, Forastiere AA, Jacobs J, Campbell BH, Saxman SB, Kish JA, Kim HE, Cmelak AJ, Rotman M et al (2004) Postoperative concurrent radiotherapy and chemotherapy for high-risk squamous-cell carcinoma of the head and neck. N Engl J Med 350(19):1937–1944

15. Cooper JS, Zhang Q, Pajak TF, Forastiere AA, Jacobs J, Saxman SB, Kish JA, Kim HE, Cmelak AJ, Rotman M et al (2012) Long-term follow-up of the RTOG 9501/intergroup phase III trial: postoperative concurrent radiation therapy and chemotherapy in high-risk squamous cell carcinoma of the head and neck. Int J Radiat Oncol Biol Phys 84(5):1198–1205

16. Ko EC, Genden EM, Misiukiewicz K, Som PM, Kostakoglu L, Chen CT, Packer S, Kao J (2012) Toxicity profile and clinical outcomes in locally advanced head and neck cancer patients treated with induction chemotherapy prior to concurrent chemoradiation. Oncol Rep 27(2):467–474

17. Vokes EE, Stenson K, Rosen FR, Kies MS, Rademaker AW, Witt ME, Brockstein BE, List MA, Fung BB, Portugal L et al (2003) Weekly carboplatin and paclitaxel followed by concomitant paclitaxel, fluorouracil, and hydroxyurea chemoradiotherapy: curative and organ-preserving therapy for advanced head and neck cancer. J Clin Oncol 21(2):320–326

18. Posner MR, Hershock DM, Blajman CR, Mickiewicz E, Winquist E, Gorbounova V, Tjulandin S, Shin DM, Cullen K, Ervin TJ et al (2007) Cisplatin and fluorouracil alone or with docetaxel in head and neck cancer. N Engl J Med 357(17):1705–1715

19. Cohen EEW, Karrison T, Kocherginsky M, Huang CH, Agulnik M, Mittal BB, Yunus F, Samant S, Brockstein B, Raez LE et al (2012) DeCIDE: a phase III randomized trial of docetaxel (D), cisplatin (P), 5-fluorouracil (F) (TPF) induction chemotherapy (IC) in patients with N2/N3 locally advanced squamous cell carcinoma of the head and neck (SCCHN). J Clin Oncol 30(15s):abstr 5500

20. Ang K, Zhang Q, Rosenthal DI, Nguyen-Tan F, Wheeler RH, Sherman EJ, Weber RS, Galvin JM, Schwartz DL, El-Naggar AK et al (2011) A randomized phase III trial (RTOG 0522) of concurrent accelerated radiation plus cisplatin with or without cetuximab for stage III-IV head and neck squamous cell carcinomas (HNC). J Clin Oncol 29(15s):abstr 5500

21. Urban D, Corry J, Rischin D (2014) What is the best treatment for patients with human papillomavirus-positive and -negative oropharyngeal cancer? Cancer 120(10):1462–1470

22. Hafkamp HC, Manni JJ, Haesevoets A, Voogd AC, Schepers M, Bot FJ, Hopman AH, Ramaekers FC, Speel EJ (2008) Marked differences in survival rate between smokers and nonsmokers with HPV 16-associated tonsillar carcinomas. Int J Cancer 122(12):2656–2664

23. Goldenberg D, Begum S, Westra WH, Khan Z, Sciubba J, Pai SI, Califano JA, Tufano RP, Koch WM (2008) Cystic lymph node metastasis in patients with head and neck cancer: an HPV-associated phenomenon. Head Neck 30(7):898–903

24. Huang SH, O'Sullivan B, Xu W, Zhao H, Chen DD, Ringash J, Hope A, Razak A, Gilbert R, Irish J et al (2013) Temporal nodal regression and regional control after primary radiation therapy for N2-N3 head-and-neck cancer stratified by HPV status. Int J Radiat Oncol Biol Phys 87(5):1078–1085
25. Ang KK, Harris J, Wheeler R, Weber R, Rosenthal DI, Nguyen-Tan PF, Westra WH, Chung CH, Jordan RC, Lu C et al (2010) Human papillomavirus and survival of patients with oropharyngeal cancer. N Engl J Med 363(1):24–35
26. O'Sullivan B, Huang SH, Siu LL, Waldron J, Zhao H, Perez-Ordonez B, Weinreb I, Kim J, Ringash J, Bayley A et al (2013) Deintensification candidate subgroups in human papillomavirus-related oropharyngeal cancer according to minimal risk of distant metastasis. J Clin Oncol 31(5):543–550
27. Chao KS, Ozyigit G, Blanco AI, Thorstad WL, Deasy JO, Haughey BH, Spector GJ, Sessions DG (2004) Intensity-modulated radiation therapy for oropharyngeal carcinoma: impact of tumor volume. Int J Radiat Oncol Biol Phys 59(1):43–50

Hypopharyngeal Cancer

8

Erkan Topkan, Berna Akkus Yildirim, Cem Parlak, and Ugur Selek

Overview

Incidence, Etiology, and Epidemiology

Hypopharyngeal carcinoma (HC) represents 7–8 % of all head and neck cancers (HNC). Tumor distribution in hypopharynx may vary by geography and gender, but in general, the most common tumor location is the pyriform sinus (75 %) followed by posterior pharyngeal wall (20 %) and postcricoid area (5 %). Patients are typically 55–70 year-old malnourished males with history of heavy tobacco and/or alcohol use, with a male/female ratio of 3–5/1. Patients with HC commonly present with sore throat, dysphagia or odynophagia with significant weight loss, hoarseness, referred otalgia, and uni- or bilateral neck mass. Primary risk factors are excessive use of tobacco and alcohol. Human papillomavirus-16 staining is positive in approximately 19 % of all HC. Plummer-Vinson syndrome is associated with postcricoid area cancers in relatively younger women.

Pathological and Biological Features

Histologically, predominating the poorly differentiated tumors, squamous cell carcinoma accounts for more than 95 % of all HC. Submucosal extension should essentially be anticipated in all HC, an extension of tumor 10 mm or

E. Topkan, MD (✉) • B.A. Yildirim, MD • C. Parlak, MD
Department of Radiation Oncology, Baskent University, Faculty of Medicine, Adana, Turkey
e-mail: drerkantopkan@yahoo.com

U. Selek, MD
Department of Radiation Oncology, Koc University, Faculty of Medicine,
Nisantasi, Istanbul, Turkey

Department of Radiation Oncology, University of Texas MD Anderson Cancer Center,
Houston, TX, USA

© Springer International Publishing Switzerland 2015
M. Beyzadeoglu et al. (eds.), *Radiation Therapy for Head and Neck Cancers:*
A Case-Based Review, DOI 10.1007/978-3-319-10413-3_8

beyond the visible lesion being not uncommon. Field tumorigenesis, submo-
cosal spread, and p53 mutations are common findings in HC. Mutations in
p53 gene are present in 75 % of cases, and the presence of disruptive mutations is strongly associated with significantly poorer survival outcomes.
Presentation with multiple tumors is not uncommon, and the risk of second
primary tumor is estimated as 25 % during the course of disease.

Definitive Therapy
Tumor localization and extension, age, performance and excessive weight
loss status, extent of lymphatic involvement, the presence of distant metastasis, anticipated functional outcome, and patient's preference are required to be
considered in the management of HC. Either surgical or nonsurgical treatment
selection for HC should favor the laryngeal preservation without any anticipated decrease in locoregional control and survival outcomes. In early-stage
disease, radiotherapy (RT) and conservative surgery are equally effective
treatment options for medically fit patients. For patients with locoregionally
advanced disease, concurrent chemoradiotherapy (CRT) is the standard of
care for organ and function preservation, total laryngopharyngectomy ± partial esophagectomy being indicated for patients not amenable for conservative
approach or salvage surgery. Cisplatin-based induction chemotherapy followed by RT or CRT may be an alternative for patients planned to undergo
total laryngopharyngectomy.

Adjuvant Therapy
Adjuvant RT or CRT is indicated in patients with postsurgical risk factors
such as close or positive margins, multiple lymph node involvement,
and/extracapsular extension (ECE). All medically fit patients without clinic or
metabolic response must be managed with salvage surgery.

1   Case Presentation

A 42-year-old male who has 20 pack-year history of smoking and 20 cc per day
alcohol consumption history with no significant past medical history presented with
voice change for 2 months and dysphagia for nearly 4 months.

His ear and nose examination revealed normal findings. He had some dental
problems requiring periodontal treatment. There are no lesions of the gingiva, buccal mucosa, floor of the mouth, oral tongue, base of the tongue, hard palate, soft
palate, tonsillar fossa, or posterior oropharyngeal wall by visualization or palpation.
On laryngoscopic examination, there was an ulcerovegetative lesion in the right
pyriform sinus behind the right arytenoids, involving its medial, anterior, and lateral
walls, fixated to the right vocal cord and in the right pyriform sinus. The left vocal
cord was mobile with no evidence of disease. There were palpable lymph nodes in
the right upper neck, and the greatest of which was measured not bigger than 2 cm.

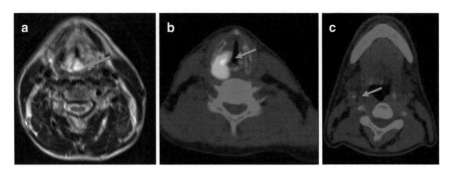

Fig. 8.1 Diagnostic images demonstrating a $30 \times 22 \times 17$ mm lesion originating from the right pyriform sinus and invading the larynx (*arrow*) through the arytenoid cartilage (**a**, magnetic resonance imaging; **b**, FDG-positron emission tomography). Right level 2 lymph node (*arrow*) demonstrated by FDG-PET (**c**)

Laryngeal CT, MRI, and PET/CT defined a protruding hypermetabolic lesion measuring 22×17 mm in axial plane and 30 mm in craniocaudal plane at the level of the right glottis filling the right pyriform sinus extending to the right arytenoid cartilage (Fig. 8.1). There were multiple hypermetabolic lymph nodes in the right level 2A, 2B, and 3, and the greatest of which was measured 14×8 mm.

A biopsy was performed from the right pyriform sinus lesion confirming the moderately differentiated squamous cell carcinoma. He was staged as T3N2bM0 (stage IVA) hypopharyngeal cancer.

2   Evidence-Based Treatment Approaches

Main prognostic factor tailoring the treatment for hypopharyngeal cancer (HC) is the disease stage (Table 8.1). Other factors include age (elderly poor), gender (male poor), tumor location (pyriform sinus apex, postcricoid region, and two- or three-wall tumors poor), and size and number of involved nodes (multiple and N3 poor) [1–3]. Definitive RT or partial laryngopharyngectomy (open or endoscopic) plus ipsi- or bilateral neck dissection (ND) are the equally effective treatment options for T1N0 and selected T2N0 patients. Salvage surgery and ND are indicated in patients with clinical or metabolic residual disease following definitive RT. In surgically treated patients with adverse features, re-resection or adjuvant therapy is indicated. For patients with ECE $\pm$ positive margins, CRT is the standard of care (category 1). In patients with positive margins, re-resection or adjuvant RT is indicated, and CRT must be considered for only T2 tumors. For patients with other risk factors, adjuvant RT or CRT must be considered.

Induction chemotherapy is the recommended treatment option for T1–T2 N+ and T3N0–N3 patients, and further treatment is determined by the response, namely, complete (CR), partial (PR), and less than PR (<PR). If CR is achieved at primary site with improved or stable disease in the neck, definitive RT (category 1) or CRT (category 2B) are the current recommendations.

Table 8.1 Staging for hypopharyngeal carcinoma (AJCC 7th edition)

Primary tumor (T)		Regional lymph node (N[b])		Distant metastasis (M)	
Tis	Carcinoma in situ	NX	Regional lymph nodes cannot be assessed	M0	No distant metastasis
T1	Tumor limited to one subsite of hypopharynx and 2 cm or less in the greatest dimension	N0	No regional lymph node metastasis	M1	Distant metastasis
T2	Tumor invades more than one subsite of hypopharynx or an adjacent site, or measures more than 2 cm but not more than 4 cm in the greatest dimension without fixation of the hemilarynx	N1	Metastasis in a single ipsilateral lymph node, 3 cm or less in the greatest dimension		
T3	Tumor more than 4 cm in the greatest dimension or with fixation of the hemilarynx or extension to the esophagus	N2	Metastasis in a single ipsilateral lymph node, more than 3 cm but not more than 6 cm in the greatest dimension, or in multiple ipsilateral lymph nodes, none more than 6 cm in the greatest dimension, or in bilateral or contralateral lymph nodes, none more than 6 cm in the greatest dimension		
T4a	Moderately advanced local disease. Tumor invades thyroid/cricoid cartilage, hyoid bone, thyroid gland, or central compartment soft tissue[a]	N2a	Metastasis in a single ipsilateral lymph node more than 3 cm but not more than 6 cm in the greatest dimension		
T4b	Very advanced local disease. Tumor invades prevertebral fascia, encases carotid artery, or involves mediastinal structures	N2b	Metastasis in multiple ipsilateral lymph nodes, none more than 6 cm in the greatest dimension		
		N2c	Metastasis in bilateral or contralateral lymph nodes, none more than 6 cm in the greatest dimension		
		N3	Metastasis in a lymph node more than 6 cm in the greatest dimension		

[a]Central compartment soft tissue includes prelaryngeal strap muscles and subcutaneous fat
[b]*Note*: Metastases at level VII are considered regional lymph node metastases

Patients with < PR at primary disease site with improved or stable disease in neck after induction chemotherapy are treated with either CRT (category 2B) or surgery. Salvage surgery is indicated if residual disease exists after CRT. RT is indicated in patients treated with surgery and no evident adverse factors. Patients with ECE and/or positive margins should undergo CRT (category 1). If other adverse factors exist, RT or CRT should be considered.

Surgery is the recommended up-front treatment for T2N+, T3N0–N3, and T1N+ patients with < PR at primary disease site after induction chemotherapy, and further treatment is determined by the status of adverse factors. If no adverse factor exists, RT is recommended. The presence of ECE and/or positive margins is an indication for CRT (category 1). If other adverse factors exist, RT or CRT should be considered.

Patients with T4a and N0–N3 should preferentially be treated with surgery followed by RT or CRT. However, induction chemotherapy followed by RT/CRT (surgery reserved for salvage), and definitive CRT is another treatment option with category 3 evidence. Postsurgical use of RT/CRT or salvage surgery after CRT is determined by the status of adverse factors. Salvage surgery and ND are indicated in patients with clinical or metabolic residual disease following CRT. Surgically treated patients with ECE and/or positive margins should undergo CRT (category 1). If other adverse factors exist, RT or CRT should be considered. Patients with progressive disease should be treated with CRT (category 2B) or surgery depending on the choice of initial treatment modality.

As a general rule, the treatment of choice is the one that proves the highest locoregional tumor control with the highest chance for preservation of respiration, deglutition, and phonation functions. In cases with T1–T2 N0 disease, both the conservative surgery and RT have similar efficacy. Vocal cord fixation by pyriform sinus tumor via invasion of the larynx portends relatively poorer outcome with definitive RT. Large nodal mass in the neck impacts the need for combination of surgery followed by RT for higher cure chance compared to either modality alone.

Type of primary resection may vary from partial laryngopharyngectomy to extremely aggressive laryngopharyngoesophagectomy and adjacent structures if involved. In addition to primary tumor resection, surgical treatment includes at least unilateral ND which is followed by RT or CRT. Conservative surgery is contraindicated in patients with:

- Vocal cord paralysis
- Transglottic extension
- Cartilage invasion
- Postcricoid invasion
- Pyriform apex invasion
- Extension beyond larynx

For small T1 and T2 lesions, 66–70 Gy RT alone may control tumor in nearly 65 % of all patients (Table 8.2).

Table 8.2 Comparative outcomes for hypopharyngeal cancer treated with radiotherapy versus surgery

Author	T stage	Patients (N)	Treatment	Local control (%)	Locoregional control (%)	5-year survival (%)
Mendenhall et al. [4]	T1–T2	35	RT	74	–	60
	T3–T4	15	RT	27	–	23
	T1–T2	6	S + RT	67	–	33
	T3–T4	47	S + RT	72	–	30
Dubois et al. [5]	T1–T2	61	RT	74	54	11
	T3–T4	148	RT	35	13	2
	T1–T2	54	S + RT	63	43	37
	T3–T4	100	S + RT	46	32	30
Van den Bogaert et al. [6]	T3–T4	66	RT	22	–	18
	T3–T4	22	S + RT	51	–	18
Pingree et al. [7]	Stages 1–2	78	RT	–	–	41
	Stages 3–4	168	RT	–	–	12
	Stages 1–2	46	S + RT	–	–	40
	Stages 3–4	285	S + RT	–	–	32
Slotman et al. [8]	T3–T4	22	RT	–	64	22
	T3–T4	32	S + RT	–	97	22

As postoperative pharyngeal or cutaneous healing is delayed by preoperative high-dose RT (60–66 Gy), to prevent or minimize postoperative complications, a dose of 45–50 Gy is recommended if RT is used in neoadjuvant setting. High-dose RT (60–66 Gy) is better tolerated when administered postoperatively with a healing period of at least 4 weeks. However, if no contraindication exists, postoperative RT should commence between 4 and 6 weeks postoperatively for better locoregional control. For aryepiglottic fold and pyriform sinus tumors, combined surgery and postoperative RT proves higher rates of 5-year disease-free and overall survival rates compared to RT or surgery alone [3].

Results of nonrandomized series demonstrated that it was possible to the spare larynx in 40–65 % patients (with/without locoregional and survival advantage) treated with induction chemotherapy followed by high-dose RT (65–75 Gy) compared to surgery followed by RT [4–8]. Based on these promising outcomes, EORTC 24891 (the European Organization for Research and Treatment of Cancer Head and Neck Cooperative Group) conducted a phase 3 randomized trial of the larynx preservation [9, 10]. This study enrolled 202 patients with locally advanced hypopharyngeal cancer (pyriform sinus or hypopharyngeal aspect of aryepiglottic fold), whose treatment would be necessitated total laryngectomy to one of two arms: arm

Table 8.3 EORTC 24891 hypopharynx/larynx preservation study [9, 10]

	Chemotherapy+RT	Surgery+RT
Randomized (N)	103	99
Eligible (n)	100	94
Primary		
Aryepiglottic fold	22 (22 %)	20 (21 %)
Pyriform sinus	78 (78 %)	74 (79 %)
Stage		
2	7 (7 %)	6 (6 %)
3	59 (59 %)	51 (54 %)
4	34 (34 %)	37 (39 %)
T3–T4	78 (78 %)	78 (83 %)
N2–N3	31 (31 %)	31 (33 %)
Complete response by T stage		
Overall	54 %	–
2	82 %	–
3	48 %	–
4	0 %	–
Survival		
Median	44 months	25 months
Disease-free (3-year/5-year)	43/%/25 %	32 %/27 %
Overall (3-year/5-year)	57 %/30 %	43 %/35 %
Larynx preservation (5-year)	35 %	–
Complete responders (5-year)	64 %	–

Abbreviations: EORTC the European Organization for Research and Treatment of Cancer, *RT* radiotherapy

A, total laryngectomy and partial pharyngectomy followed by adjuvant RT ($n=99$), and arm B, 2–3 cycles of induction cisplatin/5-fluorauracil followed by 70 Gy RT (7 weeks) in patients with complete response. Complete response was defined as total return of laryngeal mobility and macroscopic disappearance of gross tumor. Complete response was achieved in 54 % cases enrolled to induction chemotherapy arm. Complete response rates were observed to be significantly associated with T stage. At a median follow-up of 51 months (3–106 months), there was no statistically significant difference between arms A and B in terms of local (88 % vs. 83 %; $p>0.05$) and regional (81 % vs. 77 %; $p>0.05$) control rates. However, distant metastasis-free survival rates were significantly higher in arm B (64 % vs. 75 %; $p=0.04$). As depicted in Table 8.3, median and 3-year survival rates were favoring induction chemotherapy arm, but this survival advantage disappeared at 5 years. Considering the larynx preservation, the larynx was maintained in 42 and 35 % patients at 3- and 5-year time points.

Although not specific to HC, results of randomized studies and meta-analysis demonstrated that concurrent CRT is associated with superior survival rates compared to RT alone or induction chemotherapy followed by RT [11, 12]. Cisplatin is the current backbone of concurrent chemotherapy either as a single agent or combination regimen. Therefore, platinum-based concurrent CRT is widely accepted as the standard of care for locally advanced HC like other head and neck primaries.

Common to any other head and neck tumor, IMRT is the preferred technique of RT with advantages of sparing neighboring normal tissues and structures of critical importance, allowing safer escalation of the dose beyond traditional limits [13]. However, it is crucial to follow available guidelines during contouring process to prevent geographic misses and/or overtly large unnecessary radiation portals while using IMRT.

3   Target Volume Determination and Delineation Guidelines

Gross Tumor Volume (GTV)

GTV can be divided into two parts: GTV-primary (GTV_P) and GTV-nodal (GTV_N). GTV_P should include all gross disease and its visible extensions on physical examination and/or imaging studies. All nodes: >1 cm on short axis, with necrotic center, and/or positive on PET imaging should be included in GTV_N. Combination of GTV_P and GTV_N can be subscripted with the prescribed dose as a single GTV such as GTV_{70}, which is a commonly practiced dose.

Clinical Target Volume (CTV)

Based on risk definitions, there needs to be 3 CTV volumes for definitive RT/CRT as described below and depicted in Table 8.4:

- *CTV_{70}:* Due to risk for microscopic disease spread, CTV_{70} should cover GTV_{70} with a margin of 5 mm at all directions, but may be reduced to as low as 1 mm in close proximity of critical structures. For suspicious nodes, such as ≤1 cm, a separate CTV_{66} may be considered.
- *$CTV_{59.4}$:* It should encompass the entire CTV_{70} with at least 1-cm margin including the entire hypopharynx and adjacent superior and inferior structures. This volume should cover potential microscopic mucosal and submucosal disease spread. The whole larynx, adjacent fat spaces such as the preepiglottic fat, and prevertebral fascia should also be covered in this high-risk region. For lymph node regions, the CTV_{70} should be covered with a 3–5-mm margin respecting the critical structures as outlined above. Ipsilateral levels Ib-4 and lateral retropharyngeal lymph nodes should be covered in all patients. Ipsilateral level V should be covered in the presence of any gross lymph node at levels II–IV. In midline tumors such as postcricoid region and posterior pharyngeal wall, same levels should be contoured bilaterally. Retropharyngeal lymph nodes should be contoured up to the carotid canal entrance at the skull base for N1–N3 necks.

Table 8.4 Suggested CTVs to be included in radiotherapy portal in definitive and postoperative IMRT settings

CTV	Postoperative IMRT (intermediate-risk)	Postoperative IMRT (high risk)	Definitive IMRT (RT or CRT)
CTV1	Surgical bed[a]	Surgical bed[a]	Gross tumor + margins
	Residue tumor (−)	Residue tumor (−)	Primary tumor and local extensions
	Soft tissue involvement (−)	Soft tissue involvement (+)	Any enlarged node(s)
	ECE (−)	ECE (+)	
CTV2	Elective nodal regions	Elective nodal regions	Adjacent regions to CTV1
			Soft tissue
			Nodal regions
CTV3	–	–	Elective nodal regions

Abbreviations: CTV clinical target volume, *ECE* extracapsular extension, *IMRT* intensity-modulated radiotherapy, *RT* radiotherapy, *CRT* chemoradiotherapy
[a]In postoperative cases with residual tumor or nodal mass, residual mass(es) should be defined as GTV, and cases should be treated similar with definitive IMRT patients if no further surgery is planned or technically not possible

Retrostyloid space should also be covered by $CTV_{59.4}$ to encompass the upper level 2 nodes. Paratracheal and superior mediastinal lymph nodes should be covered in cases with postcricoid involvement of lower hypopharyngeal cancers.

- CTV_{54}: For N0 disease, CTV_{54} should encompass levels II–IV and retropharyngeal nodes. However, in the presence of involved contralateral node(s), ipsilateral N0 neck should also be considered high risk. For N1–N2a disease contralateral level II may end just at the level where the posterior belly of the digastric muscle crosses over the internal jugular vein. In a similar fashion, the retropharyngeal lymph node contouring may be terminated at C1 vertebrae level.

Planning Target Volume (PTV)

PTV is extra margin around the CTVs to compensate for the intra- and inter-fraction variability, uncertainties of treatment setup, and internal organ motion. It is better for any institutions to define their own PTV margin. If the institution has not performed a study to define the appropriate magnitude of PTV, following recommendations can be followed:

- PTV_{70}: As the hypopharyngeal structures are highly mobile, it is appropriate to cover CTV_{70} (primary) with 1-cm margin or more with respect to the spinal cord tolerance limits. Nodal part of PTV_{70} should be contoured with a margin of 3–5 mm around nodal part of CTV_{70}.

- $PTV_{59.4}$: It should be contoured with a margin of 3–5 mm around $CTV_{59.4}$.
- PTV_{54}: It should be contoured with a margin of 3–5 mm around CTV_{54}.

Level Definition Tips

Submandibular gland and jugular vein interface separates levels IB (submandibular) and IIa; level II (subdigastric-jugulodigastric) follows the jugular vein to the fossa; the hyoid and cricoid define the borders of levels II–III (mid-jugular) and IV (low jugular and supraclavicular); posterior edge of sternocleidomastoid defines level V (posterior cervical).

Case Contouring (Fig. 8.2)

- Check coverage of all the postcricoid region and posterior and lateral walls of hypopharynx.
- Check coverage the whole larynx from the hyoid bone to lower border of cricoid cartilage.
- Check coverage of the prevertebral fascia.
- Check coverage of the preepiglottic fat space.
- Check coverage of retropharyngeal lymph nodes up to the carotid canal at the level of the skull base.
- Check coverage of the paratracheal and superior mediastinal lymph nodes for lower hypopharyngeal tumors.
- Check coverage of level V (trapezius muscle) posteriorly.

4   Treatment Planning

- *Guidelines for Target Volume Doses:* To minimize dose to the critical structures, particularly the parotid glands, IMRT (preferred) or 3D-RT is recommended. This is critical especially when oropharyngeal structures are included in radiation portal. Typical recommended doses of RT for definitive RT/CRT and postoperative settings are described in Table 8.5. Dose distribution of PTV_{70}, $PTV_{59.4}$, and PTV_{54} Gy and related dose-volume histogram for the case presented here are demonstrated in Figs. 8.3 and 8.4, respectively.
- *Guidelines for Normal Tissue Constraints:* Normal tissue dose constraints detailed below should strictly be obeyed to prevent debilitating late toxicities. Dose-volume histogram of critical organ doses for the present representative patient is demonstrated in Fig. 8.4.

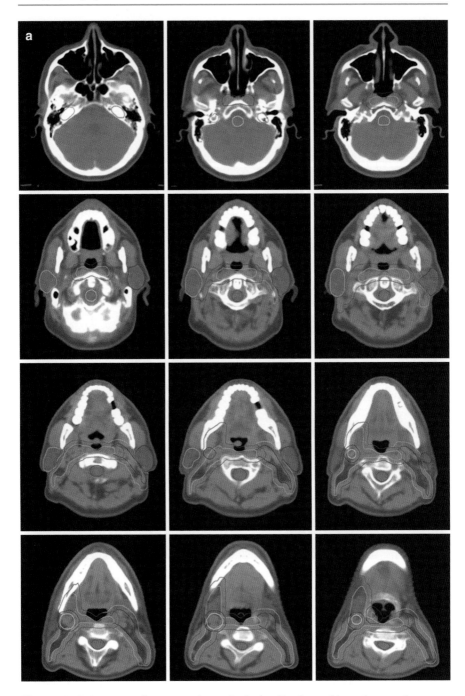

Fig. 8.2 (**a**, **b**) Representative target volumes for the locally advanced hypopharyngeal case presented here

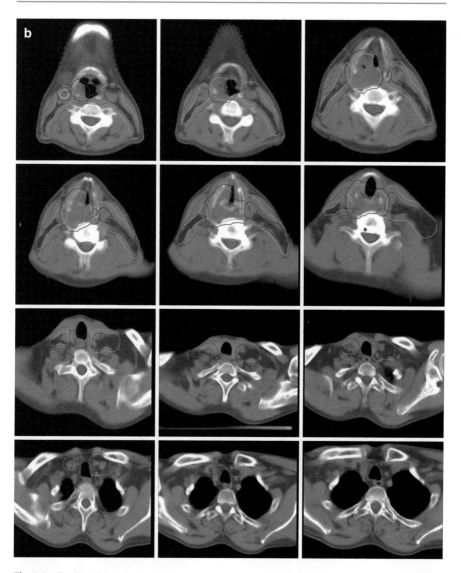

Fig. 8.2 Continued

- Parotid Glands: Mean dose (D_{mean}) of ≤ 26 Gy or less (should be achieved in at least one gland) or at least 20 cc of the combined volume of both glands should receive <20 Gy or at least 50 % of one parotid gland should receive <30 Gy.
- Brain Stem: Maximum dose (D_{max}) ≤ 54 Gy.
- Spinal Cord: D_{max} ≤ 45 Gy.
- Oral Cavity: D_{mean} <30–35 Gy.
- Brain: D_{max} ≤ 50 Gy and any large volume of brain should receive <30 Gy.
- Optic Nerve, Optic Chiasm: D_{max} <54 Gy.

Table 8.5 Recommendations for RT doses and fractionation for target volumes with standard or simultaneous integrated boost IMRT

Treatment type	PTV1	PTV2	PTV3
Definitive RT	66–70 Gy (2–2.12 Gy/fr)	59.4–66 Gy (1.8–2 Gy/fr)	46–54 Gy (1.63–2 Gy)
Definitive CRT	66–70 Gy (2–2.12 Gy/fr)	59.4–66 Gy (1.8–2 Gy/fr)	46–54 Gy (1.63–2 Gy)
Postoperative RT			
Risk factors (+)	66–70 Gy (2–2.12 Gy/fr)	59.4–66 Gy (1.8–2 Gy/fr)	46–54 Gy (1.63–2 Gy)
Risk factors (−)	60–66 Gy (2–2.12 Gy/fr)	54–63 Gy (1.8–1.9 Gy/fr)	46–54 Gy (1.63–2 Gy)
Postoperative CRT			
Risk factors (+)	66–70 Gy (2–2.12 Gy/fr)	59.4–66 Gy (1.8–2 Gy/fr)	46–54 Gy (1.63–2 Gy)
Risk factors (−)	60–66 Gy (2–2.12 Gy/fr)	54–63 Gy (1.8–1.9 Gy/fr)	46–54 Gy (1.63–2 Gy)

Abbreviations: RT radiotherapy, *CRT* chemoradiotherapy, *IMRT* intensity-modulated radiation therapy, *PTV* planning target volume

- Lens: D_{max} is 10 Gy, and <5 Gy if achievable.
- Mandible: D_{max} <69 Gy (hot spots >70 Gy should be kept out of the mandible).
- Cochlea: No more than 5 % receives ≥55 Gy.
- Brachial Plexus: 66-Gy max dose.
  - *Treatment Planning AssessmentStep 1:* Check whether the targets are adequately covered by the prescribed dose. As a common example, recommended assessment specifications in Table 8.6 are given for typical dose prescriptions of PTV1 (PTV_{70}), PTV2 ($PTV_{59.4}$), and PTV3 (PTV_{54}). However, as various scenarios of patient presentation are possible (definitive RT, definitive CRT, postoperative RT with/without adverse factors, and postoperative CRT with/without adverse factors), all dose coverage values presented in percentages should also be used for any prescribed dose levels. As far as possible, every effort should be spent to achieve IMRT plans without any deviations. However, only for extensively large tumors and tumors in close proximity to critical structures minor deviations can be accepted for necessary assessment parameters.
- *Step 2:* The presence of a large hot spot should be carefully checked and should not be permitted for more than 20 % of PTV1 (e.g., 70 Gy) to receive ≥110 % and no more than 5 % of PTV1 to receive ≥%115 of prescribed dose, respectively.
  - *Step 3:* Normal tissue constraints should carefully be checked.
  - *Step 4:* Check whether the hot/cold spots exist in the wrong place (slide by slide looking at isodose distribution): The hot spots need to be arranged in the GTV, and it is necessary to make sure that the hot spot is not on a nerve in the CTV.

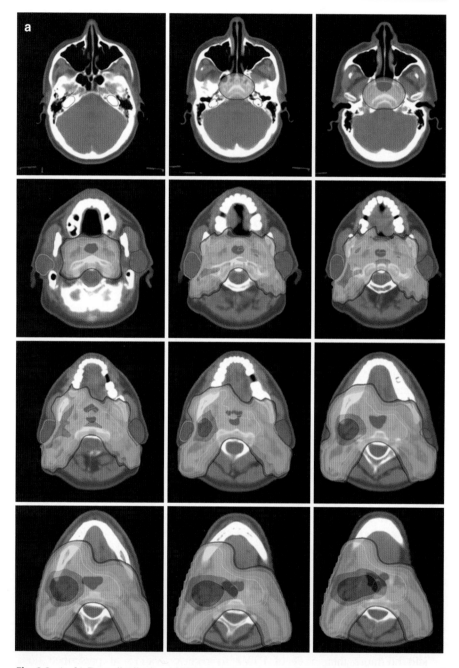

Fig. 8.3 (**a**, **b**) Dose distribution of PTV70, PTV59.4, and PTV 54 Gy for the case presented herein

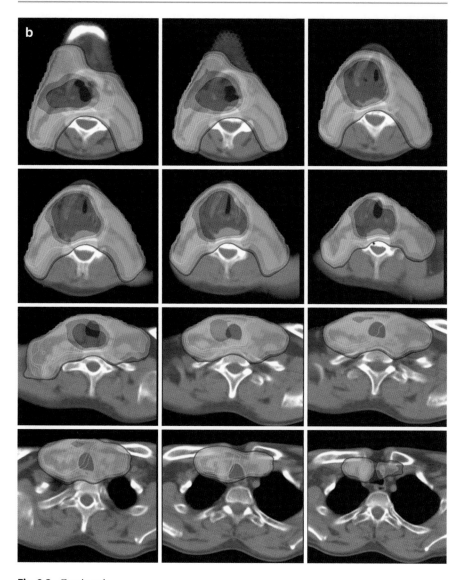

Fig. 8.3 Continued

- *Case Plan:* The patient with locally advanced hypopharyngeal carcinoma presented here was treated with concurrent CRT (cisplatin 100 mg/m^2, every 21 days) utilizing SIB-IMRT technique. As demonstrated in Figs. 8.3 and 8.4, the prescribed doses for PTV1, PTV2, and PTV3 were 70, 59.4, and 54 Gy in 33 fractions, respectively.
- *Treatment Algorithm and Patient Follow-Up:* Recommended evidence-based treatment options and patient follow-up after treatment for early- and locally advanced- stage hypopharyngeal carcinoma patients are as depicted in Figs. 8.5 and 8.6, respectively.

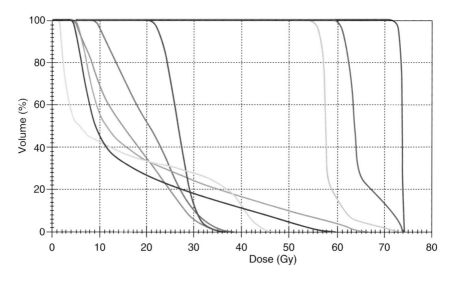

Structure	Min dose Gy	Max dose Gy	Mean dose Gy
PTV 70 Gy	70.787	74.419	73.818
PTV 59.4 Gy	57.948	74.419	66.885
PTV 54 Gy	48.583	73.891	58.474
R cochlea	4.538	38.130	16.304
L cochlea	8.512	39.890	20.620
Brain Stem	1.453	48.754	15.498
Spinal cord	18.804	37.876	26.751
R parotid	4.513	69.573	19.992
L Parotid	3.753	61.176	16.213

Fig. 8.4 Dose-volume histogram of prescribed target volume doses and critical organs at risk

Table 8.6 Specifications for IMRT plan assessment

PTV	No variation	Minor variation
PTV$_{70\,Gy}$	1. 95 % of any PTV$_{70\,Gy}$ is at or above 70 Gy	1. 95 % of PTV$_{70\,Gy}$ is at or above 70 Gy
	2. 99 % of PTV$_{70\,Gy}$ is at or above 65.1 Gy	2. 97 % of PTV$_{70\,Gy}$ is at or above 65.1 Gy
	3. No more than 20 % of PTV$_{70\,Gy}$ is at or above 77 Gy	3. No more than 40 % of PTV$_{70\,Gy}$ is at or above 77 Gy
	4. No more than 5 % of PTV$_{70\,Gy}$ is at or above 80 Gy	4. No more than 20 % of PTV$_{70\,Gy}$ is at or above 80 Gy
	5. Mean dose ≤74 Gy	5. Mean dose ≤76 Gy
PTV$_{63\,Gy}$ (if applicable)	1. 95 % of any PTV$_{63\,Gy}$ is at or above 63 Gy	1. 95 % of any PTV$_{63\,Gy}$ is at or above 58.6 Gy
	2. 99 % of PTV$_{63\,Gy}$ is at or above 58.6 Gy	2. No more than 40 % of PTV$_{63\,Gy}$ is at or above 77 Gy
	3. No more than 20 % of PTV$_{63\,Gy}$ is at or above 77 Gy	3. No more than 20 % of PTV$_{63\,Gy}$ is at or above 80 Gy
	4. No more than 5 % of PTV$_{63\,Gy}$ is at or above 80 Gy	
PTV$_{59.4\,Gy}$	1. 95 % of any PTV$_{59.4\,Gy}$ is at or above 59.4 Gy	1. 95 % of PTV$_{59.4\,Gy}$ is at or above 55.2 Gy
	2. 99 % of PTV$_{59.4\,Gy}$ is at or above 55.2 Gy	2. No more than 40 % of PTV$_{59.4\,Gy}$ is at or above 77 Gy
	3. No more than 20 % of PTV$_{59.4\,Gy}$ is at or above 77 Gy	3. No more than 20 % of PTV$_{59.4\,Gy}$ is at or above 80 Gy
	4. No more than 5 % of PTV$_{59.4\,Gy}$ is at or above 80 Gy	
PTV$_{54\,Gy}$ (if applicable)	1. 95 % of any PTV$_{54\,Gy}$ is at or above 54 Gy	1. 95 % of PTV$_{54\,Gy}$ is at or above 50.2 Gy
	2. 99 % of PTV$_{54\,Gy}$ is at or above 50.2 Gy	2. No more than 40 % of PTV$_{54\,Gy}$ is at or above 65.3 Gy
	3. No more than 20 % of PTV$_{54\,Gy}$ is at or above 65.3 Gy	3. No more than 20 % of PTV$_{54\,Gy}$ is at or above 68.3 Gy
	4. No more than 5 % of PTV$_{54\,Gy}$ is at or above 68.3 Gy	

Abbreviations: IMRT intensity-modulated radiation therapy, *PTV* planning target volume (subscript denotes for prescribed dose)

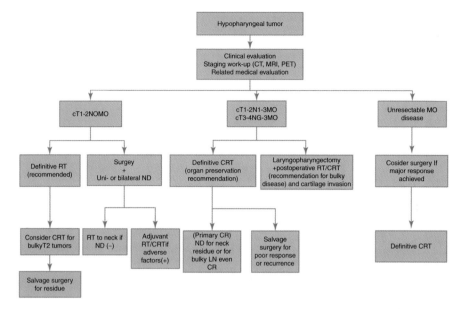

Fig. 8.5 Recommended algorithm for the treatment of hypopharyngeal cancer. *Abbreviations*: *CRT* chemoradiotherapy, *CT* computerized tomography, *LN* lymph node, *MRI* magnetic resonance imaging, *ND* neck dissection, *PET* positron emission tomography, *RT* radiotherapy

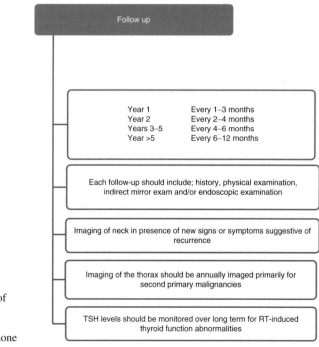

Fig. 8.6 Recommended algorithm for follow-up of hypopharyngeal cancers. *Abbreviations*: *TSH* thyroid-stimulating hormone

References

1. Farrington WT, Weighill JS, Jones PH (1986) Post-cricoid carcinoma (a ten-year retrospective study). J Laryngol Otol 100(1):79–84
2. Brugère JM, Mosseri VF, Mamelle G et al (1996) Nodal failures in patients with N0 N+ oral squamous cell carcinoma without capsular rupture. Head Neck 18(2):133–137
3. Spector JG, Sessions DG, Emami B et al (1995) Squamous cell carcinomas of the aryepiglottic fold: therapeutic results and long-term follow-up. Laryngoscope 105(7 Pt 1):734–746
4. Mendenhall WM, Parsons JT, Devine JW et al (1987) Squamous cell carcinoma of the pyriform sinus treated with surgery and/or radiotherapy. Head Neck Surg 10(2):88–92
5. Dubois JB, Guerrier B, Di Ruggiero JM et al (1986) Cancer of the piriform sinus: treatment by radiation therapy alone and with surgery. Radiology 160(3):831–836
6. Van den Bogaert W, Ostyn F, van der Schueren E (1985) Hypopharyngeal cancer: results of treatment with radiotherapy alone and combinations of surgery and radiotherapy. Radiother Oncol 3(4):311–318
7. Pingree TF, Davis RK, Reichman O, Derrick L (1987) Treatment of hypopharyngeal carcinoma: a 10-year review of 1,362 cases. Laryngoscope 97(81):901–904
8. Slotman BJ, Kralendonk JH, Snow GB et al (1994) Surgery and postoperative radiotherapy and radiotherapy alone in T3-T4 cancers of the pyriform sinus. Treatment results and patterns of failure. Acta Oncol 33(1):55–60
9. Lefebvre JL, Chevalier D, Luboinski B et al (1996) Larynx preservation in pyriform sinus cancer: preliminary results of a European Organization for Research and Treatment of Cancer phase III trial. EORTC Head and Neck Cancer Cooperative Group. J Natl Cancer Inst 88:890–899
10. Lefebvre JL, Andry G, Chevalier D et al (2012) Laryngeal preservation with induction chemotherapy for hypopharyngeal squamous cell carcinoma: 10-year results of EORTC trial 24891. Ann Oncol 23:2708–2714
11. Blanchard P, Baujat B, Holostenco V et al (2011) MACH-CH Collaborative group. Meta-analysis of chemotherapy in head and neck cancer (MACH-NC): a comprehensive analysis by tumour site. Radiother Oncol 100(1):33–40
12. Hitt R, Grau J, Lopez-Pousa A et al (2014) A randomized phase III trial comparing induction chemotherapy followed by chemoradiotherapy versus chemoradiotherapy alone as treatment of unresectable head and neck cancer. Ann Oncol 25(1):216–225
13. Lee N, Xia P, Quivey JM et al (2002) Intensity-modulated radiotherapy in the treatment of nasopharyngeal carcinoma: an update of the UCSF experience. Int J Radiat Oncol Biol Phys 53(1):12–22

Laryngeal Cancer

9

Erkan Topkan, Berna Akkus Yildirim, Cem Parlak, and Ugur Selek

Overview

Incidence, Etiology, and Epidemiology

Laryngeal carcinoma is the commonest head and neck carcinoma. Male to female ratio is around 1/5. Anatomically, larynx is situated anterior to the fourth and sixth cervical vertebrae and is divided into three regions for oncologic assessment and treatment purposes, namely, supraglottis, glottis, and subglottis. Majority of the laryngeal cancers arise from glottis followed by supra- and subglottic cancers, respectively. The strongest risk factor is the tobacco smoking, and the risk is directly associated with quantity and time of exposure. Alcohol is only second to tobacco use with its independent and synergistic actions on epithelium. Regardless of the tumor site, dysphonia and hoarseness are the commonest symptoms in laryngeal cancer patients with sore throat being the second commonest symptom in supraglottic tumors. However, besides other symptoms, a cervical mass may be the first presentation finding in some patients. Patients with hoarseness persisting longer than 3 weeks or with persisting sore throat, dysphagia, and odynophagia lasting for more than 6 weeks should be evaluated by an otolaryngologist for laryngeal carcinoma.

E. Topkan, MD (✉) • B.A. Yildirim, MD • C. Parlak, MD
Department of Radiation Oncology, Baskent University, Faculty of Medicine, Adana, Turkey
e-mail: drerkantopkan@yahoo.com

U. Selek, MD
Department of Radiation Oncology, Koc University, Faculty of Medicine, Nisantasi, Istanbul, Turkey

Department of Radiation Oncology, University of Texas MD Anderson Cancer Center, Houston, TX, USA

© Springer International Publishing Switzerland 2015
M. Beyzadeoglu et al. (eds.), *Radiation Therapy for Head and Neck Cancers: A Case-Based Review*, DOI 10.1007/978-3-319-10413-3_9

Pathological and Biological Features

More than 95 % of all laryngeal malignancies are of epithelial origin and histologically squamous cell carcinoma. Supraglottic cancers have high tendency for local invasion and uni-/bilateral cervical metastases. Depending on the tumor stage, 25–75 % of supraglottic cancers have cervical metastases at presentation, and 30 % of cN0 necks are pN+. Stage-dependent cervical metastases are rare in glottis (5–40 %) and subglottic (25–50 %). Thyroid and cricoid cartilages and associated perichondrium, conus elasticus, quadrangular membrane, and hyoepiglottic ligament are the natural barriers for laryngeal cancer spread until late stages. Two weak areas for cancer spread are anterior commissure, where thyroid membrane is deficient, and laryngeal ventricle, which is not reinforced by the quadrangular membrane.

Definitive Therapy

Age, performance, pulmonary function tests, tumor localization and extension, extent of lymphatic involvement, presence of distant metastasis, anticipated functional outcome, and patient's preference need to be considered in the management. Either surgical or nonsurgical treatment selection for laryngeal carcinoma should favor the laryngeal preservation without any anticipated decrease in locoregional control and survival outcomes. In early-stage disease, radiotherapy and conservative surgery are equally effective treatment options for medically fit patients. For patients with locoregionally advanced disease, induction chemotherapy followed by radiotherapy or concurrent chemoradiotherapy is the current standards for organ and function preservation. Doses per fraction >2 Gy should be preferred to achieve higher tumor control rates, especially in T2N0 cases.

Adjuvant Therapy

Adjuvant radiotherapy or chemoradiotherapy is indicated in patients with postsurgical risk factors such as close or positive margins, multiple lymph node involvement, and/or extracapsular extension. All medically fit patients without clinic or metabolic response must be managed with salvage surgery.

1 Case Presentation

A 67-year-old male, who has at least 150 pack year history of smoking, presented with a burning sensation in his throat and a 3-month history of right neck mass without any pain, dysphagia, odynophagia, otalgia, new voice changes, change in his cough or sputum, hemoptysis, dyspnea, aspiration, or weight loss. He had a true vocal cord benign nodule removed 20 years ago. His medical history is significant for diabetes and coronary heart disease.

His physical exam revealed normal external ear canals and tympanic membranes with appropriate light reflex. Clinical hearing acuity shows decreased to finger rub, particularly on the right side. Nasal septum was midline without deviation and was clear to anterior rhinoscopy. He is edentulous with full dentures. There are no lesions, induration, tenderness, or friability of the gingiva, buccal mucosa, floor of mouth, oral tongue, base of tongue, hard palate, soft palate, tonsillar fossa, or posterior oropharyngeal wall by visualization or palpation. Palate elevates normally. Tongue protrudes normally.

There was a 5-cm poorly mobile right level 2 conglomerate nodal mass, but no other palpable neck mass, thyroid mass, or lymphadenopathy. Cranial nerves II–XII are grossly intact without any facial numbness.

The scope was introduced into the left nasal cavity. Clearly seen was normal appearing nasopharyngeal mucosa with clearly defined bilateral Rosenmuller fossa. There was no posterior pharyngeal/oropharyngeal wall, soft palate, tonsils, vallecula, or base of tongue bulging or lesions. The scope was advanced further. The mucosa was abnormal diffusely in the larynx with nodularity on the infrahyoid laryngeal surface of the epiglottis and submucosal fullness in the region of the left false vocal cord and ventricle. The entirety of almost both true vocal cords was showing hyperkeratotic changes. The arytenoids and vocal cords were moving normally, and the airway was intact with no supraglottic edema and no accumulated secretions. The pyriformis was open. The tongue base retracted symmetrically to phonation.

His PET-CT, CT, and MRI scans defined the obvious finding as a very large conglomerate of coalesced nodal metastases measuring $5 \times 2.9 \times 5$ cm at about the hyoid level without convincing contralateral nodal metastases (Fig. 9.1). PET-CT and CT scans were negative for a definite primary, while MRI was suspicious for mucosal thickening in supraglottic area. Incidental note was made of severe atherosclerotic disease at the bifurcation with obvious stenosis of the proximal right ICA. Neck ultrasound with fine needle aspiration revealed squamous cell cancer, as well as the surgical biopsy of infrahyoid epiglottis lesion as moderately differentiated invasive squamous carcinoma.

He was staged as T2N2bM0 (stage IVA) supraglottic laryngeal squamous cell cancer.

2 Evidence-Based Treatment Approaches

2.1 Glottic Larynx

Transoral laser excision is the currently recommended treatment for carcinoma in situ, and RT is the alternative option. For T1-2N0 and selected T3N0, cases amenable for larynx preservation can be treated with radiotherapy (RT) or partial laryngectomy/endoscopic or open surgery as indicated. Persistent residue after RT should be salvaged by appropriate surgery. Patients with residual disease after surgery should undergo re-resection and/or RT/CRT (chemoradiotherapy) depending on the existence of additional adverse factors.

Patients with T3N0-1 disease requiring total laryngectomy should undergo CRT (or RT if not candidate for systemic chemotherapy) or induction chemotherapy

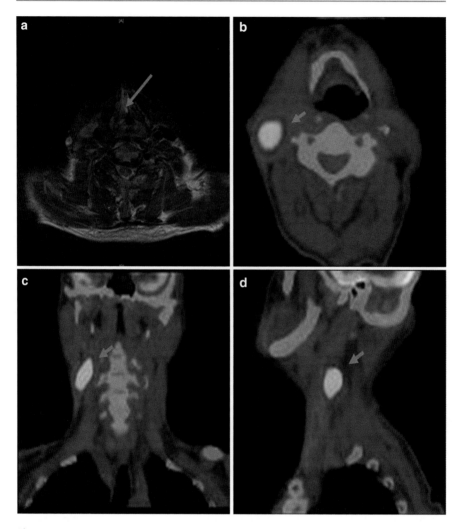

Fig. 9.1 (a) Suspicious mucosal thickening in supraglottic area on MRI. (b–d) Large conglomerate of coalesced nodal metastases measuring 5×2.9×5 cm at about the hyoid level on PET/CT images

(Category 2B) or laryngectomy with ipsilateral thyroidectomy in N0 and laryngectomy with ipsilateral thyroidectomy and ipsilateral/bilateral neck dissection (ND) in N1. Patients with complete response at primary site after RT/CRT should undergo salvage ND if residual neck disease persists. If residual disease persists at primary site, patients should undergo salvage laryngectomy and ND as indicated. In surgically treated patients with adverse features such as ECE (+) or positive margins, adjuvant CRT is indicated with category 1 evidence. RT or CRT should be considered for patients with other risk factors. Further treatment following induction chemotherapy is determined by the response at primary tumor site. Patients with complete response (CR) should receive definitive RT (Category 1). If residual neck disease persists, salvage ND should be performed as indicated. Patients with partial response (PR) at primary site should receive RT (Category 1) or CRT (Category 2B). If residue persists following RT/CRT, salvage surgery is indicated. If primary site response is < PR, surgery is indicated. In such patients, if pathologically ECE (+) or surgical margins (+), CRT is indicated (Category 1). For patients with other risk factors, RT or CRT should be considered.

Patients with T3N2-3 disease requiring total laryngectomy should be treated with either CRT, laryngectomy with ipsilateral thyroidectomy and ipsilateral/bilateral ND, or induction chemotherapy followed by adjuvant treatment determined by response. Additional treatment should be performed similar to T3N1 disease as described above.

Patients with T4aN0-3 should undergo laryngectomy with total thyroidectomy and unilateral/bilateral ND as indicated. Such patients should receive postoperative RT or CRT, observation being reserved only for highly selected patients. For selected T4a patients refusing surgery, CRT or induction chemotherapy followed by RT/CRT is recommended. Any residual neck disease should be salvaged by ND, and residual disease at primary site should further be discussed with the patient for salvage surgery and ND.

2.2   Supraglottic Larynx

T1-2 N0 and selected T3N0 cases amenable for larynx preservation can either be treated with RT or open partial supraglottic laryngectomy/endoscopic resection with/without ND. Persistent residue after RT should be salvaged by appropriate surgery. Patients with residual disease after surgery should undergo re-resection or RT (Category 1) or CRT (Category 2B) depending on the existence of additional adverse features.

Patients with T3N0-1 disease requiring total laryngectomy should undergo CRT (or RT if not candidate for systemic chemotherapy) or induction chemotherapy (Category 2B) or laryngectomy with ipsilateral thyroidectomy and ipsilateral/bilateral ND. Patients with complete response at primary site after RT/CRT should undergo salvage ND if residual neck disease persists. If residual disease persists at primary site, patients should undergo salvage laryngectomy and ND as indicated. In surgically treated patients with pN0 or only single node involvement without other adverse factors, adjuvant RT should be considered. Patients with adverse features such as ECE (+) or positive margins should undergo CRT (Category 1). RT or CRT should be considered for patients with other risk factors. Following induction chemotherapy, further treatment is determined by the response at primary tumor site. Patients with complete response (CR) at primary site should receive definitive RT (Category 1). If residual neck disease persists, salvage ND should be performed. Patients with partial response (PR) at primary site should receive RT (Category 1) or CRT (Category 2B). If residue persists following RT/CRT, salvage surgery is indicated. If primary site response is < PR, surgery is indicated. In such patients, if pathologically ECE (+) or surgical margins (+), CRT is indicated (Category 1). For patients with other risk factors, RT or CRT should be considered.

Patients amenable for organ preserving surgery with T1-2 N1-3 and selected T3N1 disease should be treated with definitive RT or CRT or partial supraglottic laryngectomy and ND or induction chemotherapy. For patients treated with RT or CRT, any residual neck disease should be salvaged by ND, and if residue persists at primary disease site, salvage surgery and ND should be considered as indicated. For surgically treated patients with ECE (+) or margins (+), CRT (Category 1) and RT/CRT for other adverse factors should be considered. Salvage treatment after induction chemotherapy should be performed as described above.

T3N2-3 patients requiring total laryngectomy should be treated with CRT, laryngectomy with ipsilateral thyroidectomy and ND, or induction chemotherapy followed by adjuvant treatment determined by response type as detailed previously. Additional treatment should be performed for either modality similar with to their T3N1 disease as described above.

T4aN0-3 patients should undergo laryngectomy with total thyroidectomy and unilateral/bilateral ND as indicated. Such patients should receive postoperative RT or CRT, observation being reserved only for highly selected patients. For selected T4a patients refusing surgery, CRT or induction chemotherapy followed by RT/CRT is recommended. Any residual neck disease should be salvaged by ND, and residual disease at primary site should further be discussed with the patient for salvage surgery and ND.

2.3   Subglottic Larynx

Subglottic tumors are exceedingly rare, accounting for only 2 % of all laryngeal cancers. Most patients present with advanced disease (T3-4 N+). Definitive RT, CRT, and surgery are treatment options for such patients. If surgery is chosen, total laryngectomy should be performed regarding the tumor location and invasion of thyroid and/or cricoid cartilages. Postoperative RT/CRT should be considered to increase locoregional control rates. Salvage surgery is indicated in any patient with residual primary or neck disease.

Stage of disease is the strongest prognostic factor for laryngeal carcinoma (Table 9.1). Among staging parameters, M-stage determines the survival, while T- and N-stage are strong predictors of local control and distant metastasis, respectively. Female patients, in general, do better than male counterparts.

Functional larynx preservation without any decrease in local control and survival rates is the ultimate goal of any treatment directed to any stage of laryngeal carcinoma.

Although stripping and RT are options for carcinoma in situ, early RT should be preferred because recurrence is frequent and hoarsening of the voice may become evident due to cord thickening after repeated stripping. Additionally, many patients with carcinoma in situ have obvious lesions that probably contain invasive carcinoma, and early RT will spare many patients from repeat biopsy and many others from unavoidable RT.

Table 9.1 American Joint Committee on Cancer staging for laryngeal carcinoma (AJCC 7th edition)

Primary tumor (T)	
Tis	Carcinoma in situ
Supraglottis	
T1	Tumor limited to one subsite of supraglottis with normal vocal cord mobility
T2	Tumor invades mucosa of more than one adjacent subsite of supraglottis or glottis or region outside the supraglottis (e.g., mucosa of base of tongue, vallecula, medial wall of pyriform sinus) without fixation of the larynx
T3	Tumor limited to larynx with vocal cord fixation and/or invades any of the following: postcricoid area, preepiglottic space, paraglottic space, and/or inner cortex of thyroid cartilage
T4a	Moderately advanced local disease: Tumor invades through the thyroid cartilage and/or invades tissues beyond the larynx (e.g., trachea, soft tissues of neck including deep extrinsic muscle of the tongue, strap muscles, thyroid, or esophagus)
T4b	Very advanced local disease: Tumor invades prevertebral space, encases carotid artery, or invades mediastinal structures
Glottis	
T1	Tumor limited to the vocal cord(s) (may involve anterior or posterior commissure) with normal mobility
T1a	Tumor limited to one vocal cord
T1b	Tumor involves both vocal cords
T2	Tumor extends to supraglottis and/or subglottis, and/or with impaired vocal cord mobility
T3	Tumor limited to the larynx with vocal cord fixation and/or invasion of paraglottic space inner cortex of the thyroid cartilage
T4a	Moderately advanced local disease: Tumor invades through the outer cortex of the thyroid cartilage and/or invades tissues beyond the larynx (e.g., trachea, soft tissues of neck including deep extrinsic muscle of the tongue, strap muscles, thyroid, or esophagus)
T4b	Very advanced local disease: Tumor invades prevertebral space, encases carotid artery, or invades mediastinal structures
Subglottis	
T1	Tumor limited to the subglottis
T2	Tumor extends to vocal cord(s) with normal or impaired mobility
T3	Tumor limited to larynx with vocal cord fixation
T4a	Moderately advanced local disease: Tumor invades cricoid or thyroid cartilage and/or invades tissues beyond the larynx (e.g., trachea, soft tissues of neck including deep extrinsic muscles of the tongue, strap muscles, thyroid, or esophagus)
T4b	Very advanced local disease: Tumor invades prevertebral space, encases carotid artery, or invades mediastinal structures
Regional lymph node (N)	
NX	Regional lymph nodes cannot be assessed
N0	No regional lymph node metastasis
N1	Metastasis in a single ipsilateral lymph node, 3 cm or less in greatest dimension
N2	Metastasis in a single ipsilateral lymph node, more than 3 cm but not more than 6 cm in greatest dimension, or in multiple ipsilateral lymph nodes, none more than 6 cm in greatest dimension, or in bilateral or contralateral lymph nodes, none more than 6 cm in greatest dimension

(continued)

Table 9.1 (continued)

Primary tumor (T)	
N2a	Metastasis in a single ipsilateral lymph node more than 3 cm but not more than 6 cm in greatest dimension
N2b	Metastasis in multiple ipsilateral lymph nodes, none more than 6 cm in greatest dimension
N2c	Metastasis in bilateral or contralateral lymph nodes, none more than 6 cm in greatest dimension
N3	Metastasis in a lymph node more than 6 cm in greatest dimension
Distant metastasis (M)	
M0	No distant metastasis
M1	Distant metastasis

From Greene [14]

Transoral laser excision and RT are options for T1 and T2 glottic tumors. As the voice quality is inversely related with the quantity of tissue removed, RT is the first choice of treatment in many centers, surgery being reserved for RT failures. Five years local control rates following RT are in the range of 85–95 % for T1 and 60–89 % for T2 tumors [1].

There is a direct association between the overall treatment time and local control rates for laryngeal carcinoma patients treated with definitive RT. Longer treatment duration related with lower dose per fraction in the range of 1.8–1.9 Gy results in poorer local control rates compared to same total doses with >2 Gy per fraction. In a prospective randomized study reported by Yamazaki et al., authors compared 2 Gy/fr ($n=89$) and 2.25 Gy/fr ($n=91$) and reported significantly higher local control rates with 2.25 Gy/fr (94 % vs. 77 %; $p=0.004$) [2].

As respective 5-year isolated neck recurrence rates are 0, 3, and 8 % for T1, T2A, and T2B patients, neck treatment is not indicated [3]. Achievement of local control is of extreme importance as neck recurrences increase up to 20–25 % in primary disease site recurrences, which may be a sign of distant metastasis and poor survival [4].

Similar with glottic cancers, early supraglottic cancers can be treated with either of transoral laser excision, open surgery, or RT. As local control and voice quality outcomes are similar many centers prefer RT as the initial management option. In a series of 274 T1-2 supraglottic larynx cancer patients treated with RT demonstrated excellent 5-year local control (T1 = 100 % vs. T2 = 86 %) and cause specific survival (T1 = 100 % vs. T2 = 93 %) rates [5].

For locally advanced laryngeal carcinoma, total laryngectomy, induction chemotherapy followed by surgery or RT/CRT, and concurrent CRT are options for treatment.

The era of larynx preservation with CRT emerged with the publication of Veterans Affairs Laryngeal Cancer Study in 1991 [6]. In this study, 332 stage III or IV laryngeal cancer patients were randomized into induction chemotherapy with cisplatin and fluorouracil followed by RT or surgery followed by RT groups.

Although overall 2-year survival rates were 68 % for both groups, larynx was preserved in 64 % of patients in the induction chemotherapy arm. Significant differences between the two groups were seen with fewer local failures in the surgery group ($p=0.0005$) and fewer distant metastases in the chemotherapy group ($p=0.016$). These results led to a shift in advanced-stage laryngeal cancer treatment toward a primary nonsurgical approach, reserving total laryngectomy for salvage.

The RTOG 91–11 study randomly compared three nonoperative approaches in the treatment of 547 patients with stage III or IV laryngeal cancer: induction chemotherapy (cisplatin and fluorouracil) followed by RT, RT given concurrently with cisplatin, and RT alone [7]. Primary aim was to determine proper timing of chemotherapy (induction vs. concurrent). At 2 years, proportion of patients maintaining an intact larynx was greatest in the concurrent CRT group (88 %), compared to the induction chemotherapy (75 %; $p=0.005$) and the RT alone groups (70 %; $p<0.001$). Locoregional control was also significantly better in the concurrent CRT group than the induction chemotherapy and RT alone group (78 % vs. 61 % vs. 56 %, respectively). Both chemotherapy arms had longer disease-free survival compared to RT alone. Other randomized studies of larynx preservation are as summarized in Table 9.2.

Based on the results of these benchmark studies, induction chemotherapy followed by RT or upfront concurrent CRT (preferred) became the standards of care for locally advanced laryngeal carcinoma

For early-stage laryngeal carcinomas, 3D-conformal RT is preferred. If necessary, bolus material of appropriate thickness should be used to involve anterior commissure in the high-dose region. For locally advanced laryngeal carcinoma patients, IMRT is the preferred technique of RT with advantage of sparing surrounding normal tissues and structures of critical importance, allowing safer escalation of the dose beyond traditional limits. However, it is crucial to follow available guidelines during contouring process to prevent geographic misses and/or overtly large unnecessary radiation portals while using IMRT.

3 Target Volume Determination and Delineation Guidelines

In patients treated with induction chemotherapy target volumes should be determined on pre-chemotherapy images. In an effort to increase the accuracy of target volume determination and to prevent geographic misses, it is better to use co-registered pre- and post-chemotherapy images during delineation.

3.1 Gross Tumor Volume (GTV)

GTV can be divided into two parts; GTV-primary (GTV_P) and GTV-nodal (GTV_N). GTV_P should include all gross disease and its visible extensions on physical examination and/or imaging studies. All nodes, >1 cm on short axis, with necrotic center, and/

Table 9.2 Randomized larynx preservation trials

Reference	Patients (N)	Treatment arms	Overall survival	Larynx preservation
VALCS [6]	332	S + RT	68 % (2-y)	–
		ICT + RT	68 % (2-y)	64 % (2-y)
RTOG-91-11 [7]	547	ICT + RT	38.5 % (10-y)	67.5 % (10-y)
		CCRT	27.5 % (10-y)	81.7 % (10-y)
		RT alone	31.5 % (10-y)	63.8 % (10-y)
EORTC 24891 [8]	202	S + RT	32.6 % (5-y)	–
		ICT + RT	13.8 % (10-y)	–
			38 % (5-y)	21.9 (5-y)
			13.1 % (10-y)	8.7 % (10-y)
GETTEC [9]	68	S + RT	84 % (2-y)	–
		ICT + RT	69 % (2-y)	42 % (2-y)
GORTEC 2000–2001 [10]	213	ICT (PF) + RT	60 % (3-y)	57.5 % (3-y)
		ICT (TPF) + RT	60 % (3-y)	70.3 %) (3-y)
TAX 324 (Subgroup) [11]	166	ICT (PF) + CCRT	40 % (3-y)	32 % (3-y)
		ICT (TPF) + CCRT	57 % (3-y)	52 % (3-y)
EORTC 24954 [12]	450	Sequential PF + RT	62.2 % (3-y)	39.5 % (3-y)
		Alternating PF + RT	48.5 % (5-y)	30.5 % (5-y)
			64.8 % (3-y)	45.4 % (3-y)
			51.9 % (5-y)	36.2 % (5-y)
TREMPLIN [13]	153	ICT (TPF) + CCRT (Platin based)	92 % (18 mo)	87 % (18 mo)
		ICT (TPF) + CCRT (Cetuximab)	89 % (18 mo)	82 % (18 mo)

Abbreviations: CCRT concomitant chemoradiotherapy, *ICT* induction chemotherapy, *PF* cisplatin, flourouracil, *RT* radiotherapy, *TPF* docetaxel, cisplatin, fluorouracil, *S* surgery, *y* year, *mo* month

or positive on PET imaging, should be included in GTV_N. Combination of GTV_P and GTV_N can be subscripted with the prescribed dose as a single GTV such as GTV_{70}, which is a commonly practiced dose for locally advanced laryngeal carcinoma.

3.2   Clinical Target Volume (CTV)

CTV is the entire larynx from the top of thyroid notch to the bottom of the thyroid cartilage for T1-2 N0 cancers. Based on risk definitions, there needs to be 3 CTV volumes for definitive RT/CRT of locally advanced laryngeal tumors (Table 9.3):

Table 9.3 Typical target volume definitions for postoperative IMRT and definitive RT/CRT

CTV	Postoperative IMRT (intermediate risk)	Postoperative IMRT (high risk)	Definitive IMRT (RT or CRT)
CTV1	Surgical bed[a]	Surgical bed[a]	Gross tumor + margins
	Residue tumor (−)	Residue tumor (−)	Primary tumor and local extensions
	Soft tissue involvement (−)	Soft tissue involvement (+)	Any enlarged node(s)
	ECE (−)	ECE (+)	
CTV2	Elective nodal regions	Elective nodal regions	Adjacent regions to CTV1
			Soft tissue
			Nodal regions
CTV3	–	–	Elective nodal regions

Abbreviations: CRT chemoradiotherapy, *CTV* clinical target volume, *ECE* extracapsular extension, *IMRT* intensity modulated radiation therapy, *RT* radiotherapy
[a]In postoperative cases with residual tumor or nodal mass, residual mass(es) should be defined as GTV, and cases should be treated similar with definitive IMRT patients if no further surgery is planned or technically not possible

- *CTV$_{70}$:* Due to risk for microscopic disease spread, CTV$_{70}$ should cover GTV$_{70}$ with a margin of 5 mm at all directions but may be reduced to as low as 1 mm in close proximity of critical structures. For borderline nodes, such as ≤1 cm, a separate CTV$_{63-66}$ may be considered.
- *CTV$_{59.4}$:* It should encompass entire CTV$_{70}$ with at least 1-cm margin. This volume should cover potential microscopic mucosal and submucosal routes of disease spread. For lymph node regions, the CTV$_{70}$ should be covered with a 3–5 mm margin respecting the critical structures, which can be reduced to as low as 1 mm. High-risk nodal regions to be covered are levels II–IV on the involved N + neck. Level 1B should optionally be included if level 2 is positive. Level 5 is not included unless levels 2–4 are massively involved. As typical lymphatic drainage of larynx does not contain retropharyngeal nodes, they should not be included in the absence of bulky node, which may cause retrograde lymphatic flow to retropharyngeal nodes. Level 6 should be included in presence of subglottic extension or primary lesions originating from this region.
- *CTV$_{54}$:* Should include levels 2–4 of the uninvolved neck.

3.3   Planning Target Volume (PTV)

PTV is extra margin around the CTVs to compensate for the intra- and inter-fraction variabilities, uncertainties of treatment set-up, and internal organ motion. It is better for any institutions to define their own PTV margin. If the institution has not performed a study to define the appropriate magnitude of PTV, following recommendations can be followed:

- *PTV$_{70}$:* Although should be determined institutionally, as the laryngeal structures are highly mobile, it is appropriate to cover CTV$_{70}$ (primary) with 1-cm margin or more (especially in craniocaudal direction. Nodal part of PTV$_{70}$ should be contoured with a margin of 3–5 mm around nodal part of CTV$_{70}$.
- *PTV$_{59.4}$:* Should be contoured with a margin of 3–5 mm around CTV$_{59.4}$.
- *PTV$_{54}$:* Should be contoured with a margin of 3–5 mm around CTV$_{54}$.

3.4   Level definition tips are as follows

Submandibular gland and jugular vein interface separates levels 1B (submandibular) and 2a; level 2 (subdigastric-jugulodigastric) follows the jugular vein to the fossa; hyoid and cricoid define the borders of levels 2, 3 (midjugular), and 4 (low jugular and supraclavicular); and posterior edge of sternocleidomastoid defines level 5 (posterior cervical).

3.5   Case Contouring (Fig. 9.2)

- Check coverage whole larynx from the hyoid bone to lower border of cricoid cartilage.
- Check coverage prevertebral fascia.
- Check coverage of the paratracheal and prelaryngeal lymph nodes in locally advanced disease.

3.6   Guidelines for Normal Tissue Constraints

Normal tissue dose constraints detailed below should strictly be obeyed to prevent debilitating late toxicities. Dose-volume histogram of critical organ doses for the present representative patient is demonstrated in Figs. 9.3 and 9.4:
- Parotid glands: Mean dose (D$_{mean}$) of $\leq$26 Gy or less (should be achieved in at least one gland) or at least 20 cc of the combined volume of both glands should receive <20 Gy or at least 50 % of one parotid gland should receive <30 Gy).
- Brain stem: maximum dose (D$_{max}$) $\leq$54 Gy
- Spinal cord: D$_{max}$ $\leq$45 Gy
- Oral cavity: D$_{mean}$ <30–35 Gy
- Brain: D$_{max}$ $\leq$50 Gy and any large volume of brain should receive <30 Gy
- Optic nerve, Optic Chiasm: D$_{max}$ <54 Gy
- Lens: D$_{max}$ is 10 Gy, and <5 Gy if achievable
- Mandible: D$_{max}$ <69 Gy (hot spots >70 Gy should be kept out of the mandible).
- Cochlea: No more than 5 % receives $\geq$55 Gy
- Brachial plexus: 66 Gy max dose

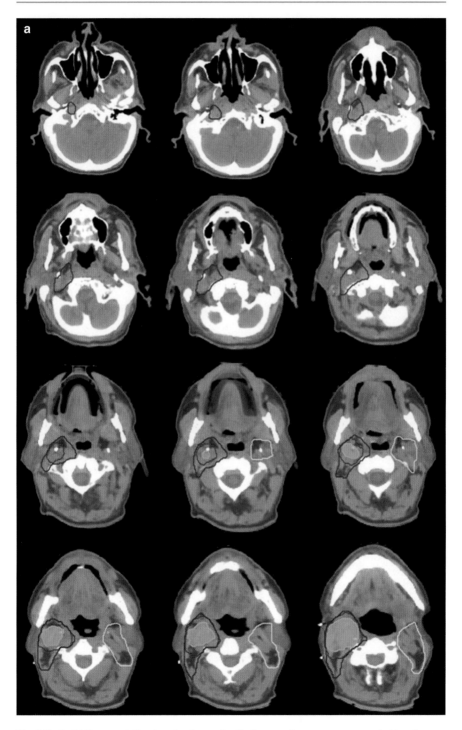

Fig. 9.2 (**a**, **b**) Representative target volumes for the laryngeal cancer case presented herein

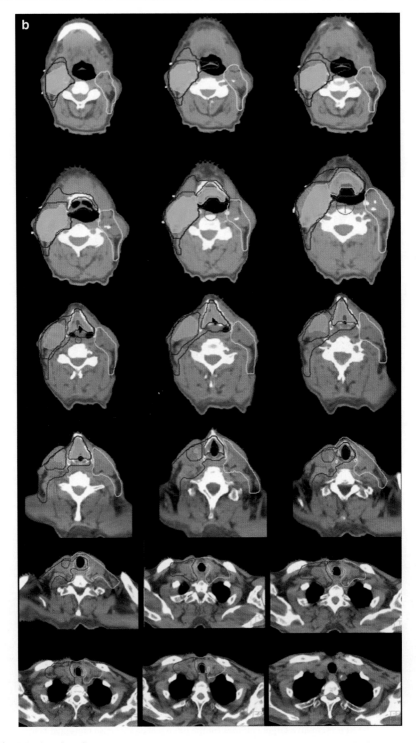

Fig. 9.2 (continued)

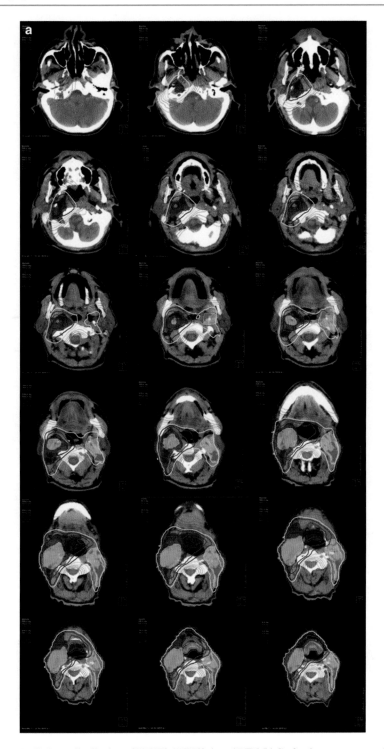

Fig. 9.3 (**a**, **b**) Dose distribution of PTV70, PTV59.4, and PTV 54 Gy for the case presented here

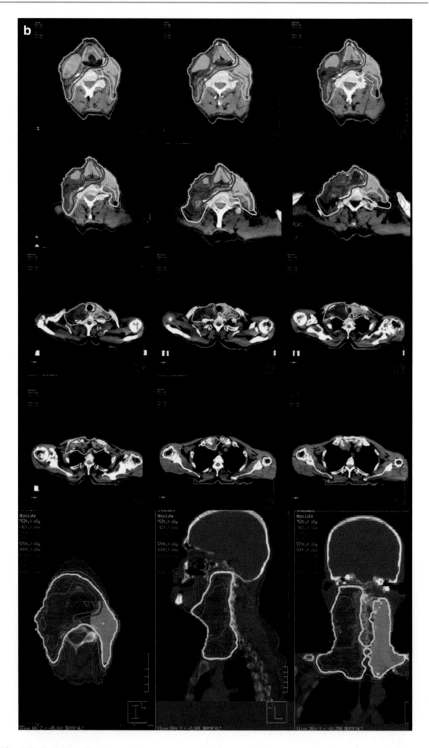

Fig. 9.3 (continued)

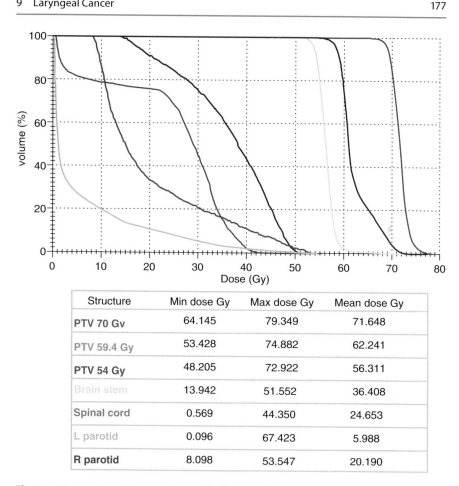

Structure	Min dose Gy	Max dose Gy	Mean dose Gy
PTV 70 Gv	64.145	79.349	71.648
PTV 59.4 Gy	53.428	74.882	62.241
PTV 54 Gy	48.205	72.922	56.311
Brain stem	13.942	51.552	36.408
Spinal cord	0.569	44.350	24.653
L parotid	0.096	67.423	5.988
R parotid	8.098	53.547	20.190

Fig. 9.4 Dose-volume histogram of prescribed target volume doses and critical organs at risk

4 Treatment Planning Assessment

- *Step 1:* Check whether the targets are adequately covered by prescribed dose for PTV1, 2, and 3 according to Table 9.4. As far as possible, every effort should be spent to achieve IMRT plans without any deviations. However, only for extensively large tumors and tumors in close proximity to critical structures, minor deviations can be accepted for necessary assessment parameters.
- *Step 2:* Presence of a large hot spot should be carefully checked and should not be permitted for more than 20 % of PTV1 (e.g., 70 Gy) to receive ≥110 % and no more than 5 % of PTV1 to receive ≥%115 of prescribed dose, respectively.
- *Step 3:* Normal tissue constraints should carefully be checked.
- *Step 4:* Check whether the hot/cold spots exist in the wrong place (slide by slide by looking at isodose distribution): The hot spots needs to be arranged in the GTV. It is necessary to make sure that the hot spot is not on a nerve in the CTV.

Table 9.4 Criteria for IMRT plan assessment

PTV	No variation	Minor variation
PTV70	1. 95 % of any PTV70 is at or above 70 Gy	1. 95 % of PTV70 is at or above 70 Gy
	2. 99 % of PTV70 is at or above 65.1 Gy	2. 97 % of PTV70 is at or above 65.1 Gy
	3. No more than 20 % of PTV70 is at or above 77 Gy	3. No more than 40 % of PTV70 is at or above 77 Gy
	4. No more than 5 % of PTV70 is at or above 80 Gy	4. No more than 20 % of PTV70 is at or above 80 Gy
	5. Mean dose ≤74 Gy	5. Mean dose ≤76 Gy
PTV63 (if applicable)	1. 95 % of any PTV63 is at or above 63 Gy	1. 95 % of any PTV63 is at or above 58.6 Gy
	2. 99 % of PTV63 is at or above 58.6 Gy	2. No more than 40 % of PTV63 is at or above 77 Gy
	3. No more than 20 % of PTV63 is at or above 77 Gy	3. No more than 20 % of PTV63 is at or above 80 Gy
	4. No more than 5 % of PTV63 is at or above 80 Gy	
PTV59.4	1. 95 % of any PTV59.4 is at or above 59.4 Gy	1. 95 % of PTV59.4 is at or above 55.2 Gy
	2. 99 % of PTV59.4 is at or above 55.2 Gy	2. No more than 40 % of PTV59.4 is at or above 77 Gy
	3. No more than 20 % of PTV59.4 is at or above 77 Gy	3. No more than 20 % of PTV59.4 is at or above 80 Gy
	4. No more than 5 % of PTV59.4 is at or above 80 Gy	
PTV54 (if applicable)	1. 95 % of any PTV54 is at or above 54 Gy	1. 95 % of PTV54 is at or above 50.2 Gy
	2. 99 % of PTV54 is at or above 50.2 Gy	2. No more than 40 % of PTV54 is at or above 65.3 Gy
	3. No more than 20 % of PTV54 is at or above 65.3 Gy	3. No more than 20 % of PTV54 is at or above 68.3 Gy
	4. No more than 5 % of PTV54 is at or above 68.3 Gy	

IMRT intensity modulated radiotherapy, *PTV* planning target volume

Case plan: The patient with locally advanced hypopharyngeal carcinoma presented here was treated with concurrent CRT (cisplatin 100 mg/m^2, every 21 days) utilizing SIB-IMRT technique. As demonstrated in Figs. 9.3 and 9.4, the prescribed doses for PTV1, PTV2, and PTV3 were 70, 59.4, and 54 Gy in 33 fractions, respectively.

Treatment algorithm and patient follow-up: Recommended-evidence based treatment options and patient follow-up after treatment for early and locally advanced-stage hypopharyngeal carcinoma patients are as depicted in Figs. 9.5, 9.6, 9.7, 9.8, 9.9, 9.10 and 9.11, respectively.

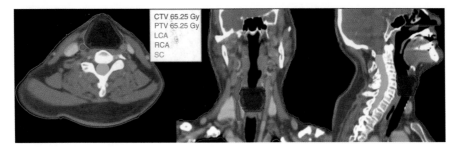

Fig. 9.5 Target volumes and critical organ contours for early-stage (T1-2 N0) laryngeal carcinoma on axial (**a**), coronal (**b**), and sagittal (**c**) planes (*CTV* clinical target volüme, *LCA* left carotid artery, *PTV* planning target volume, *RCA* right carotid artery, *SC* spinal cord)

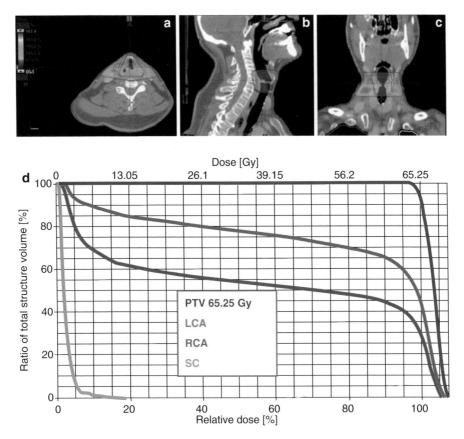

Fig. 9.6 Dose coverages (**a–c**) and dose-volume histogram (**d**) for 3D-conformal plans for early stage laryngeal cancer case

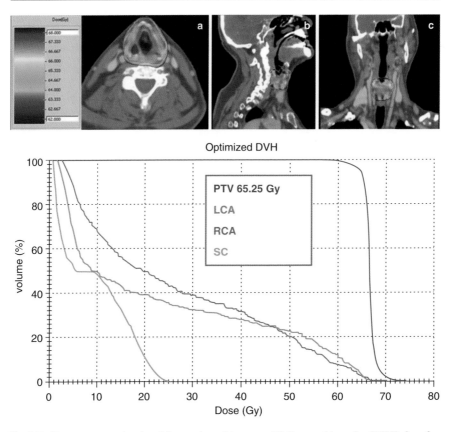

Fig. 9.7 Dose coverages (**a–c**) and dose-volume histogram (**d**) for carotid sparing IMRT plans for early-stage laryngeal cancer case

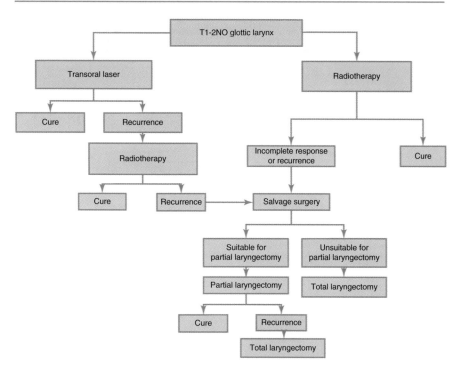

Fig. 9.8 Recommended algorithm for treatment of early glottic laryngeal cancer

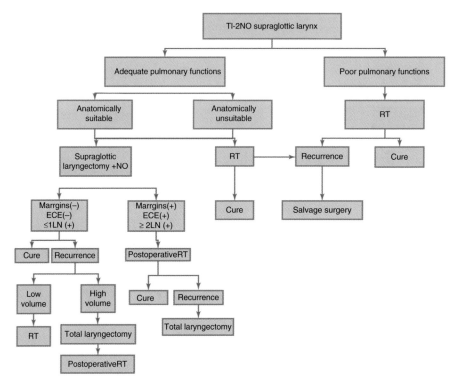

Fig. 9.9 Recommended algorithm for treatment of early supraglottic laryngeal cancer. *Abbreviations:* *ECE* extracapsular extension, *LN* lymph node, *ND* neck dissection, *RT* radiotherapy

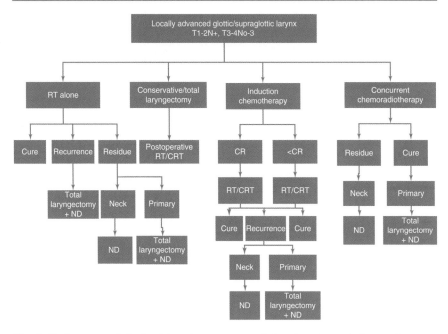

Fig. 9.10 Recommended algorithm for treatment of locally advanced laryngeal cancer. *Abbreviations*: *CR* complete response, *CRT* chemoradiotherap, *ECE* extracapsular extension, *LN* lymph node, *ND* neck dissection, *RT* radiotherapy

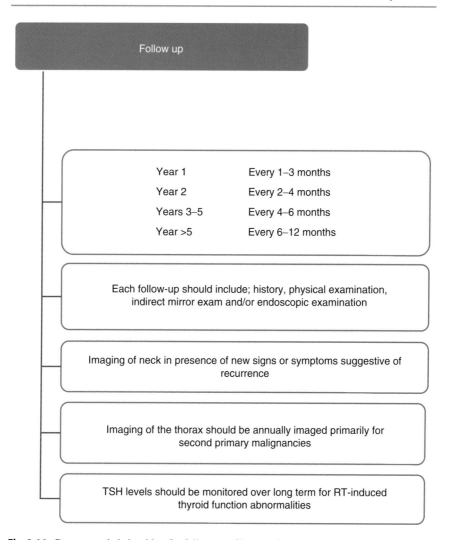

Fig. 9.11 Recommended algorithm for follow-up of laryngeal cancers

References

1. Tomeh C, Holsinger FC (2014) Laryngeal cancer. Curr Opin Otolaryngol Head Neck Surg 22(2):147–153
2. Yamazaki H, Nishiyama K, Tanaka E et al (2006) Radiotherapy for early glottic carcinoma (T1N0M0): results of prospective randomized study of radiation fraction size and overall treatment time. Int J Radiat Oncol Biol Phys 64(1):77–82
3. Mendenhall WM, Amdur RJ, Morris CG et al (2001) T1-T2N0 squamous cell carcinoma of the glottic larynx treated with radiation therapy. J Clin Oncol 19(20):4029–4036
4. Mendenhall WM, Werning JW, Hinerman RW et al (2004) Management of T1-T2 glottic carcinomas. Cancer 100(9):1786–1792
5. Hinerman RW, Mendenhall WM, Amdur RJ et al (2002) Carcinoma of the supraglottic larynx: treatment results with radiotherapy alone or with planned neck dissection. Head Neck 24(5):456–467
6. The Department of Veterans Affairs Laryngeal Cancer Study Group (1991) Induction chemotherapy plus radiation in patients with advanced laryngeal cancer. N Engl J Med 324(24):1685–1690
7. Forastiere AA, Zhang Q, Weber RS et al (2013) Long-term results of RTOG 91–11: a comparison of three nonsurgical treatment strategies to preserve the larynx in patients with locally advanced larynx cancer. J Clin Oncol 31:845–852
8. Lefebvre JL, Andry G, Chevalier D et al (2012) Laryngeal preservation with induction chemotherapy for hypopharyngeal squamous cell carcinoma: 10-year results of EORTC trial 24891. Ann Oncol 23:2708–2714
9. Richard JM, Sancho-Garnier H, Pessey JJ et al (1998) Randomized trial of induction chemotherapy in larynx carcinoma. Oral Oncol 34:224–228
10. Pointreau Y, Garaud P, Chapet S et al (2009) Randomized trial of induction chemotherapy with Cisplatin and 5-Fluorouracil with or without Docetaxel for Larynx Preservation. J Natl Cancer Inst 101:498–506
11. Posner MR, Norris CM, Wirth LJ et al (2009) Sequential therapy for the locally advanced larynx and hypopharynx cancer subgroup in TAX 324: survival, surgery, and organ preservation. Ann Oncol 20:921–927
12. Lefebvre JL, Rolland F, Tesselaar M et al (2009) Phase 3 randomized trial on larynx preservation comparing sequential vs alternating chemotherapy and radiotherapy. J Natl Cancer Inst 101:142–152
13. Lefebvre JL, Pointreau Y, Rolland F et al (2013) Induction chemotherapy followed by either chemoradiotherapy or bioradiotherapy for larynx preservation: the TREMPLIN Randomized Phase II Study. J Clin Oncol 31:853–859
14. Greene FL, American Joint Committee on Cancer, American Cancer Society (2010) AJCC cancer staging manual, 7th edn. Springer, New York

Salivary Gland

10

Melis Gultekin, Sezin Yuce Sari, Gokhan Ozyigit,
Mustafa Cengiz, Gozde Yazici, Pervin Hurmuz,
and Murat Beyzadeoglu

Overview

Epidemiology

There are three major salivary glands as pairs: parotid, submandibular, and sublingual glands. Besides, many minor glands are located mainly in the upper aerodigestive tract but also in the palate, buccal mucosa, base of tongue, pharynx, trachea, cheek, lip, gingiva, floor of mouth, tonsil, paranasal sinuses, nasal cavity, and nasopharynx. Malignant tumors of salivary glands comprise less than 0.5 % of all cancers and constitute less than 5 % of all head and neck cancers [1]. The majority of tumors (both benign and malignant) arise in the parotid glands; however, when it comes to malignant tumors only, parotid glands have the lowest incidence comparing to smaller glands [2, 3]. The benign tumors mostly occur in younger patients and female sex, where the malignant ones are equally distributed in both sexes but are seen in older population.

Low intake of vitamins A and C, heavy smoking, irradiation, occupational exposure to beauty or hair products were shown to be contributed in the development of salivary gland tumors [4–7].

M. Gultekin, MD (✉) • S.Y. Sari, MD • G. Ozyigit, MD
M. Cengiz, MD • G. Yazici, MD • P. Hurmuz, MD
Department of Radiation Oncology, Hacettepe University,
Faculty of Medicine,
Sihhiye, Ankara, Turkey
e-mail: melisbahadir@yahoo.com

M. Beyzadeoglu, MD
Department of Radiation Oncology, Gulhane Military Medical School, Etlik, Ankara, Turkey

© Springer International Publishing Switzerland 2015
M. Beyzadeoglu et al. (eds.), *Radiation Therapy for Head and Neck Cancers:
A Case-Based Review*, DOI 10.1007/978-3-319-10413-3_10

Pathological and Biological Features

Histopathologically, salivary gland tumors may be divided into benign and malignant forms. Benign tumors are called adenomas and consist of pleomorphic adenoma (most common), Warthin tumor (second most common), myoepithelioma, oncocytoma, types of papilloma, and types of cystadenoma. Malignant tumors include mucoepidermoid carcinoma (most common pathology of the parotid glands), acinic cell carcinoma (second most common of the parotid glands), adenoid cystic carcinoma (most common in other major and minor salivary glands), adenocarcinoma, cystadenocarcinoma, mucinous adenocarcinoma, oncocytic carcinoma, myoepithelial carcinoma, and more uncommon types of SCC, small cell carcinoma, salivary duct carcinoma, lymphoma, undifferentiated carcinoma, and etc. Salivary gland carcinomas are graded as low or high grade.

Definitive Therapy

Surgery is the mainstay of treatment, followed by radiotherapy (RT) in high-risk patients. In locally advanced, unresectable, and recurrent tumors, RT may be the primary treatment. Neutron therapy was reported to be more efficacious compared to photons in terms of local control (LC).

Adjuvant Therapy

In order to increase LC, radiation therapy is performed for unfavorable prognostic factors such as T3-4 tumors, close or positive surgical margins, high grade, bone or base of skull invasion, perineural invasion, or recurrent tumor. Adjuvant chemotherapy has not shown to be effective.

1   Case Presentation

A 63-year-old male applied with left facial nerve paralysis, presenting for nearly 7 months. There was no response to steroids. In his second attack of paralysis, he also felt numbness in the lower part of the left side of his face. He had a history of social alcohol consumption for nearly 40 years but no cigarette smoking.

His physical examination revealed left facial nerve paralysis with all branches being totally paralytic. The movements of the soft palate, oral tongue, and eye were normal. Nasal septum was deviated to the left. He had posterior laryngitis, but the oral cavity, oropharynx, and hypopharynx were normal. Cervical lymphadenopathy was not detected.

The MRI revealed a 2.9 × 2.2 cm lesion in the intersection of deep and superficial lobes of the left parotid gland (Fig. 10.1). There were also lymphadenopathies in levels Ib–III of the left side of the neck seen on PET-CT scan (Fig. 10.2).

The histologic evaluation of the fine-needle aspiration of the left parotid was reported as a high-grade salivary gland carcinoma.

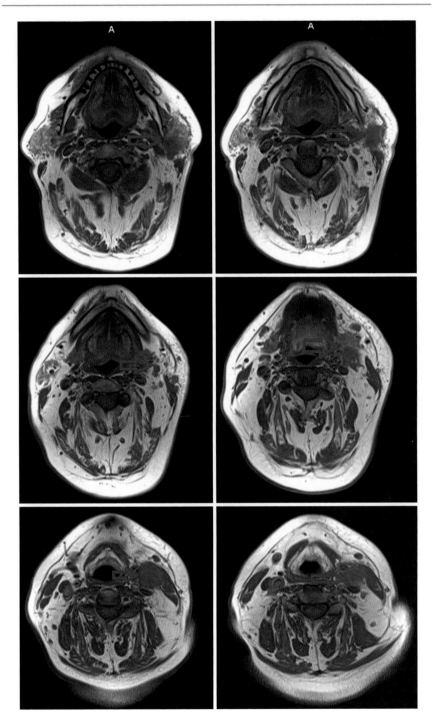

Fig. 10.1   MRI revealed a 2.9×2.2 cm lesion in the intersection of deep and superficial lobes of the left parotid gland, as well as lymphadenopathies in levels Ib, II, and III. *Red arrows* showing the primary lesion and pathological neck nodes

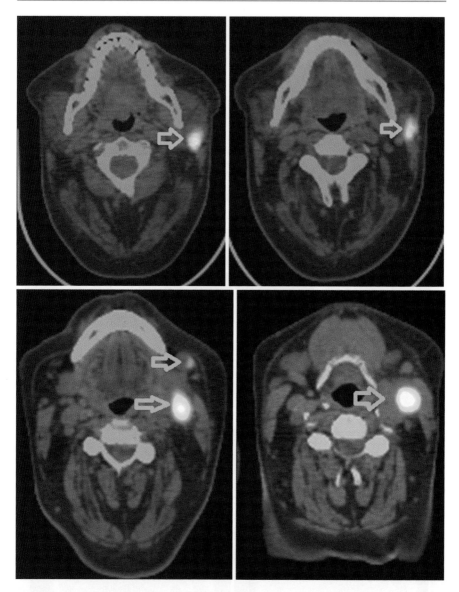

Fig. 10.2 Lymphadenopathies in levels Ib, II, and III of the left side of the neck seen on PET-CT scan. *Blue arrows* showing FDG uptake in pathological neck nodes

After facial nerve decompression, radical parotidectomy with modified radical neck dissection of left side was performed. The pathology revealed salivary duct carcinoma, coherent with sarcomatoid component. The tumor was 3 cm in size. Surgical margins were positive in anterior and posterior margins as well as the margin over facial nerve. Out of 40 resected lymph nodes, 6 were metastatic, and ECE was positive.

The patient was staged as T2N2bM0 parotid gland cancer.

2   Evidence-Based Treatment Approaches

Unless the nerve is involved, facial nerve-preserving surgery with adjuvant radiation therapy (RT) is the preferred treatment. More aggressive surgery has not been shown to increase local control (LC). Adjuvant RT does not have any negative effect on the function of the facial nerve [8]. In patients with clinically positive lymph nodes, neck dissection should be performed prior to adjuvant RT [9]. However, in case of high-risk factors for local recurrence (LR), where adjuvant RT is indicated postoperatively, neck treatment can be performed solely with RT [10, 11]. Exception to this is patients with parotid tumors with facial nerve involvement, submandibular tumors, or tumors of minor salivary glands in the floor of mouth, tongue, pharynx, and larynx, in whom elective nodal dissection of levels I–III is the standard treatment [10].

Several studies reported LC rates that ranged between 51 and 99 % and 5- and 10-year overall survival (OS) rates up to 78 and 67 %, respectively, with different treatment modalities. In patients treated with surgery alone, high rates of LR have been reported [3]. Retrospective studies showed that adjuvant RT improves LC, particularly in cases with locally advanced disease, positive lymph nodes, close or positive surgical margins, bone invasion, or PNI [9, 12–16].

Dose-response relationship was reported for photons [9], and a minimum dose of 66 Gy is recommended. Neutron therapy was shown to result in higher LC rates in unresectable and recurrent tumors. However, late complications were also higher and survival rates were equal with neutrons compared to photons [17–19].

Pleomorphic adenomas are benign tumors, and superficial parotidectomy is the standard treatment with high rates of LC [20]. Radiotherapy is indicated in case of positive surgical margins, recurrent and unresectable tumors [21–24]. Adenoid cystic carcinomas are known for their late recurrences [15]. Simple excision is not adequate for these tumors, as residual tumor is highly probable. Fortunately, nodal recurrence risk is relatively low. Combined treatment strategies yield high LC rates [13, 25–28]. Salivary duct carcinoma is highly aggressive; therefore, all cases should receive adjuvant RT. The surgical approach for most minor salivary gland tumors is more difficult; thus adjuvant RT is indicated nearly in all cases.

Sublingual gland tumors are mostly locally advanced and high grade but have a low propensity for lymph node involvement. Adjuvant RT is indicated in the majority of the patients as they are mostly high risk.

Chemotherapy (CT) is used for palliative treatment only [29]. There are limited data regarding the efficacy of concurrent adjuvant chemoradiotherapy (CRT). In patients with T3–4 tumors, positive surgical margins, positive lymph nodes, or PNI, CRT was shown to have a LC rate higher than 90 %, but the number of patients was limited and severe acute toxicity was reported [30, 31]. In another study where 24 patients were evaluated, postoperative CRT was found to be superior to RT alone in terms of OS [32].

3   Target Volume Determination and Delineation Guidelines

Gross Tumor Volume (GTV)

GTV should include the gross tumor and involved lymph nodes detected by clinical examination, CT, MRI, PET/CT, and intraoperative findings, if operated. GTV is divided into two; GTVp defines the primary tumor, and GTVn defines the involved lymph nodes. In postoperative cases GTV is not stated as it is assumed to be no tumor or grossly involved lymph nodes left.

Following structures should be evaluated carefully whether they are involved in parotid tumors:

- *Anteriorly:*Is the skin involved?
  - *Laterally:*Is the skin involved?
  - Are the pterygoid plates intact?
    - *Medially:*Is there tumor extension into the mandible?
    - Is the masseter muscle involved?
- Posteriorly:
  - Does the tumor extend to the stylohyoid foramen which the facial nerve passes through?
  - Is there tumor extension through the ear canal?
  - Is the carotid artery intact?
    - *Superiorly:*Is the skull involved?
      - *Inferiorly:*Is there extraparenchymal extension?

Clinical Target Volume (CTV)

- *CTV1* includes the entire ipsilateral parotid gland, parapharyngeal space, infratemporal fossa, and ipsilateral subdigastric nodes. It is not necessary to treat the surgical scar to full skin dose as scar failure is less than 1 %. In case of PNI, the cranial nerve pathway from the parotid up to the base of the skull should also be delineated.
- *CTV2* covers the entire operative bed as it is the region of high risk for subclinical disease and potential routes of spread.
- *CTV3* is the low-risk regions of subclinical disease. For parotid tumors, elective neck irradiation is indicated in patients with locally advanced disease, squamous and undifferentiated histologies, facial nerve involvement at diagnosis, and recurrence. Ipsilateral levels Ib, II, and III should be treated. Bilateral elective neck irradiation is not recommended. In case of positive lymph nodes after neck dissection, ipsilateral neck between level I and IV should be included. For submandibular tumors, elective ipsilateral levels I–IV should be treated. If the tumor

extends toward the midline, bilateral neck irradiation is indicated. Elective neck irradiation is not necessary in small acinic cell and adenoid cystic cancers. Delineation of the cranial nerve pathway also is not required in adenoid cystic carcinomas of submandibular gland with focal PNI as the recurrence rate of this site is very low with a risk of significant morbidity; however, this is not the case for minor salivary gland adenoid cystic carcinomas. The base of skull also is included in tumors of the palate and paranasal sinuses. Elective neck irradiation is indicated for tumors of the tongue, floor of the mouth, pharynx, and larynx. Lingual and hypoglossal nerves may also be invaded in sublingual tumors. In this case, the pathway from the gland to the skull base should be delineated as well.

Planning Target Volume (PTV)

A margin of 3–5 mm is added in all directions; however, it may be minimized to 1 mm in areas adjacent to critical structures.

Case Contouring

Case contouring is demonstrated in Fig. 10.3.

4   Treatment Planning

- *Guidelines for Target Volume Doses:* Guidelines for target volume doses are summarized in Table 10.1.
- *Guidelines for Normal Tissue Constraints:* Guidelines for normal tissue constraints are summarized in Table 10.2.
- *Treatment Planning Assessment* (Figs. 10.4 and 10.5)
  - *Step 1:* Check whether the targets are adequately covered: All plans should be normalized to at least 95 % of the volume of PTV60 is covered by the 60 Gy isodose surface and 99 % of PTV60 needs to be at or above 56 Gy. It is confusing to evaluate all PTV DVHs, and one may end up slight underdosing of PTV2 and PTV3 when a uniform 3 mm margin is added, which is generally 80 % coverage of PTV2 and PTV3 mostly due to critical structure sparing. However, if your nodal CTVs are relatively generous including some muscle outside of the nodal fat plane, much of the setup error is "built in" to the CTV contour drawn, so some physicians only evaluate CTV2 and CTV3 by looking at dose distributions on the treatment plan and not PTV DVH. It is very important to evaluate the DVH of PTV1, because a very tight margin on CTV1 could result in underdosing of gross disease due to daily setup error. Be careful to ensure that PTV1 should receive at least >90 % of prescribed dose.

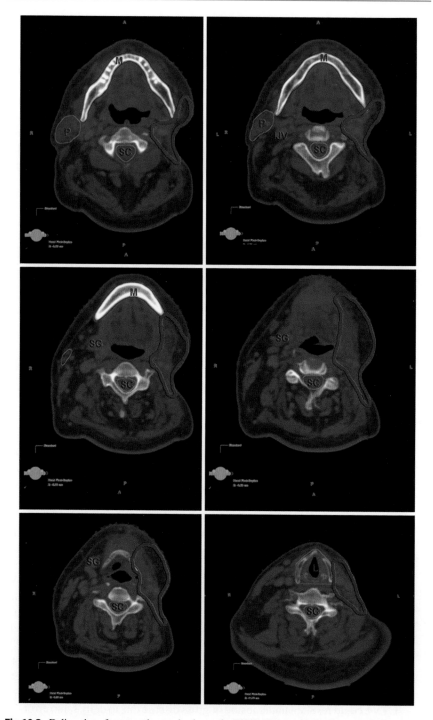

Fig. 10.3 Delineation of target and normal volumes for T2N2bM0 parotid gland cancer (CTV$_{64\,Gy}$=red)

Table 10.1 Guidelines for target volume doses

TNM	CTV1 (60 Gy/30 fr)	CTV2 (54 Gy/30 fr)	CTV3 (50 Gy/30 fr)
T1–2 N0	GTVp (whole gland)	–	–
T3–4 N0	GTVp (whole gland)	0.5 cm	Ipsilateral Ib–III and intraparotidal except for adenoid cystic and acinic cell carcinomas
T1–4 N+	GTVp (whole gland), GTVn	Ipsilateral adjacent lymph nodes (intraparotidal, the one level above, and the one level below)	Remaining lymph nodes (ipsilateral Ib–IV, contralateral I–III for submandibular tumors extending toward midline)

Table 10.2 Guidelines for normal tissue constraints

Structure	Constraints
Brain	Mean <50 Gy
	For larger volumes, <30 Gy
Brain stem	Maximum <54 Gy (no more than 1 % to exceed 60 Gy)
Spinal cord	Maximum <45 Gy (no more than 1 % to exceed 50 Gy)
Eyes	Maximum <50 Gy
Lenses	Maximum <10 Gy, try to achieve 5 Gy (as low as possible)
Optic nerves	<50 Gy (maximum 54 Gy)
Optic chiasm	<50 Gy (maximum 54 Gy)
Parotid glands	Mean of one gland <26 Gy or 50 % volume of one gland <30 Gy or 20 cc of both glands <20 Gy
Submandibular and sublingual glands	As low as possible
Each cochlea	Volume receiving 55 Gy <5 %
Mandibula and temporomandibular joint	Maximum <70 Gy, (no more than 1 cc to exceed 75 Gy)
Oral cavity (excluding PTVs)	Mean <30–40 Gy,
	No hot points receiving >60 Gy in oral cavity region
Lips	Mean <20 Gy,
	Maximum <30 Gy
Esophagus, postcricoid pharynx	Mean <45 Gy
Glottic larynx	Mean <45 Gy
Brachial plexus	Maximum <66 Gy

– *Step 2:* Check whether there is a large hot spot: No more than 20 % of PTV60 is at or above 66 Gy, and no more than 5 % of PTV60 is at or above 68.5 Gy.
– *Step 3:* Check whether the normal tissue constraints are met.

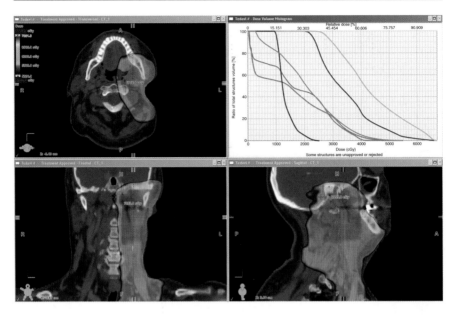

Fig. 10.4 Sagittal, coronal and axial sections of IMRT plan for T2N2bM0 parotid gland cancer

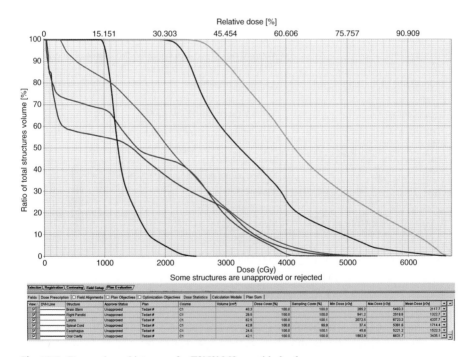

Fig. 10.5 Dose volume histogram for T2N2bM0 parotid gland cancer

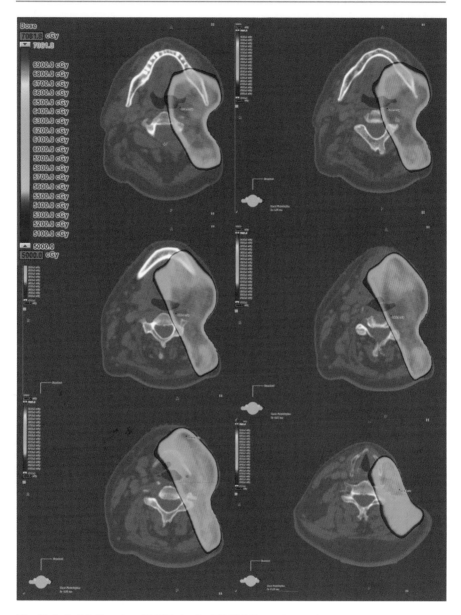

Fig. 10.6   Serial slices from IMRT plan for T2N2bM0 parotid gland cancer

- *Step 4:* Check whether the hot/cold spots exist in the wrong place (slide by slide looking at isodose distribution): The hot spots need to be arranged in the GTV, and it is necessary to make sure that the hot spot is not on a nerve in the CTV.

- *Case Plan:* The case presented here was treated with IMRT as shown in Fig. 10.6. Surgical bed as $CTV_{66 Gy}$ was prescribed 66 Gy since there was surgical margin positivity; left level I–III were irradiated as $CTVn_{64 Gy}$ and received 64 Gy due to extracapsular nodal extension; left level IV and SCF as $CTVn_{57 Gy}$ received 57 Gy. Cisplatin was given with a weekly dose of 40 mg/m².
- *Treatment Algorithm*

T1-2, N0, M0
Surgery (in case of high-grade tumor, close or + surgical margin or subtotal excision, + lymph nodes, deep lobe involvement in parotid tumors, facial nerve involvement, or PNI add adjuvant RT)
If unresectable; RT
No role for chemotherapy
T3-4, ≥N1, M0
Surgery + adjuvant RT
If unresectable; RT
No demonstrated role of chemotherapy

- *Follow-up:* Every 3 months for the first 2 years, every 4–6 months for years 3–5, and then annually. Complete remission through clinical examination and imaging studies are necessary. Distinguish viable residual or slowly regressing tumor or post-therapy changes by MRI and PET/CT

References

1. Terhaard CJH (2013) Salivary glands. In: Halperin EC, Perez AC, Brady LW (eds) Principles and practice of radiation oncology. Lippincott Williams & Wilkins, Philadelphia, p 778
2. Jones AS et al (1998) Tumours of the minor salivary glands. Clin Otolaryngol Allied Sci 23(1):27–33
3. Spiro RH (1986) Salivary neoplasms: overview of a 35-year experience with 2,807 patients. Head Neck Surg 8(3):177–184
4. Johns ME, Kaplan M (1986) Surgical therapy of tumors of the salivary glands. In: Panje WR, Thawley SE, Batsakis J et al (eds) Comprehensive management of head and neck tumors. WB Saunders, Philadelphia
5. Muscat JE, Wynder EL (1998) A case/control study of risk factors for major salivary gland cancer. Otolaryngol Head Neck Surg 118(2):195–198
6. Saku T et al (1997) Salivary gland tumors among atomic bomb survivors, 1950–1987. Cancer 79(8):1465–1475
7. Modan B et al (1998) Increased risk of salivary gland tumors after low-dose irradiation. Laryngoscope 108(7):1095–1097
8. Brown PD et al (2000) An analysis of facial nerve function in irradiated and unirradiated facial nerve grafts. Int J Radiat Oncol Biol Phys 48(3):737–743
9. Terhaard CH et al (2005) The role of radiotherapy in the treatment of malignant salivary gland tumors. Int J Radiat Oncol Biol Phys 61(1):103–111
10. Ferlito A et al (2002) Management of the neck in cancer of the major salivary glands, thyroid and parathyroid glands. Acta Otolaryngol 122(6):673–678

11. Stennert E et al (2003) High incidence of lymph node metastasis in major salivary gland cancer. Arch Otolaryngol Head Neck Surg 129(7):720–723
12. Armstrong JG et al (1990) Malignant tumors of major salivary gland origin. A matched-pair analysis of the role of combined surgery and postoperative radiotherapy. Arch Otolaryngol Head Neck Surg 116(3):290–293
13. Fu KK et al (1977) Carcinoma of the major and minor salivary glands: analysis of treatment results and sites and causes of failures. Cancer 40(6):2882–2890
14. Mendenhall WM et al (2005) Radiotherapy alone or combined with surgery for salivary gland carcinoma. Cancer 103(12):2544–2550
15. Terhaard CH et al (2004) Salivary gland carcinoma: independent prognostic factors for locoregional control, distant metastases, and overall survival: results of the Dutch head and neck oncology cooperative group. Head Neck 26(8):681–692; discussion 692–3
16. Therkildsen MH et al (1998) Salivary gland carcinomas–prognostic factors. Acta Oncol 37(7–8):701–713
17. Laramore GE et al (1993) Neutron versus photon irradiation for unresectable salivary gland tumors: final report of an RTOG-MRC randomized clinical trial. Radiation Therapy Oncology Group. Medical Research Council. Int J Radiat Oncol Biol Phys 27(2):235–240
18. Douglas JG et al (2003) Treatment of salivary gland neoplasms with fast neutron radiotherapy. Arch Otolaryngol Head Neck Surg 129(9):944–948
19. Huber PE et al (2001) Radiotherapy for advanced adenoid cystic carcinoma: neutrons, photons or mixed beam? Radiother Oncol 59(2):161–167
20. Witt RL (2002) The significance of the margin in parotid surgery for pleomorphic adenoma. Laryngoscope 112(12):2141–2154
21. Carew JF et al (1999) Treatment of recurrent pleomorphic adenomas of the parotid gland. Otolaryngol Head Neck Surg 121(5):539–542
22. Dawson AK, Orr JA (1985) Long-term results of local excision and radiotherapy in pleomorphic adenoma of the parotid. Int J Radiat Oncol Biol Phys 11(3):451–455
23. Liu FF et al (1995) Benign parotid adenomas: a review of the Princess Margaret Hospital experience. Head Neck 17(3):177–183
24. Renehan A, Gleave EN, McGurk M (1996) An analysis of the treatment of 114 patients with recurrent pleomorphic adenomas of the parotid gland. Am J Surg 172(6):710–714
25. Garden AS et al (1995) The influence of positive margins and nerve invasion in adenoid cystic carcinoma of the head and neck treated with surgery and radiation. Int J Radiat Oncol Biol Phys 32(3):619–626
26. Renehan AG et al (1999) Clinico-pathological and treatment-related factors influencing survival in parotid cancer. Br J Cancer 80(8):1296–1300
27. Simpson JR, Thawley SE, Matsuba HM (1984) Adenoid cystic salivary gland carcinoma: treatment with irradiation and surgery. Radiology 151(2):509–512
28. Storey MR et al (2001) Postoperative radiotherapy for malignant tumors of the submandibular gland. Int J Radiat Oncol Biol Phys 51(4):952–958
29. Lalami Y et al (2006) Salivary gland carcinomas, paranasal sinus cancers and melanoma of the head and neck: an update about rare but challenging tumors. Curr Opin Oncol 18(3):258–265
30. Pederson AW et al (2011) Adjuvant chemoradiotherapy for locoregionally advanced and high-risk salivary gland malignancies. Head Neck Oncol 3:31
31. Schoenfeld JD et al (2012) Salivary gland tumors treated with adjuvant intensity-modulated radiotherapy with or without concurrent chemotherapy. Int J Radiat Oncol Biol Phys 82(1):308–314
32. Tanvetyanon T et al (2009) Outcomes of postoperative concurrent chemoradiotherapy for locally advanced major salivary gland carcinoma. Arch Otolaryngol Head Neck Surg 135(7):687–692

Metastatic Cancer in Neck Node with Occult Primary

Erkan Topkan, Berna Akkus Yildirim, and Cem Parlak

Overview

Epidemiology

Metastatic cervical carcinoma of unknown primary (MCCUP) represents 3 % of all tumors and 2–9 % of all head and neck cancers (HNC). Currently, no risk factor has been identified except those defined for subsites of HNC. Patients must be evaluated for Epstein-Barr virus (EBV), human papillomavirus (HPV), and sexual behaviors, which may provide useful clues about the primary. Typically, majority of cases are 55–65 years aged males with history of chronic tobacco and/or alcohol use presenting with uni- or bilateral painless mass(es) in the upper two third neck.

Pathological and Biological Features

Histologically, squamous cell carcinoma (SCC) accounts for 53–77 % of all MCCUP followed by undifferentiated carcinomas (20 %). Other pathologies are rare, but a diagnosis of adenocarcinoma in the lower third of the neck is important as it usually denotes for a primary below the clavicles. Histologic examination of the biopsy specimen for EBV and HPV is important for tailoring the further diagnostic search and treatment plans.

Definitive Therapy

Currently, there exists no standard treatment recommendation for MCCUP. Treatment is directed by two most significant prognostic factors, namely, nodal stage (N) and status of extracapsular extension (ECE). For N1 disease and ECE (−), single-modality treatment with selective neck dissection (ND) or involved field radiotherapy (RT) is indicated. For N1 but ECE (+) and N2-3 disease, a combined approach with pre- or postoperative RT/CRT or

E. Topkan, MD (✉) • B.A. Yildirim, MD • C. Parlak, MD
Department of Radiation Oncology, Baskent University, Faculty of Medicine, Adana, Turkey
e-mail: drerkantopkan@yahoo.com

© Springer International Publishing Switzerland 2015
M. Beyzadeoglu et al. (eds.), *Radiation Therapy for Head and Neck Cancers:
A Case-Based Review*, DOI 10.1007/978-3-319-10413-3_11

upfront CRT followed by planned ND for only those without clinical/metabolic complete response is justified. For unilateral tumors, bilateral neck RT decreases the contralateral recurrences with no proven survival advantage. Similarly, despite commonly practiced, clinical impact of inclusion of pharyngeal mucosal sites in the RT portal is debated.

Adjuvant Therapy
Benefit of adjuvant or consolidation chemotherapy is uncertain but warrants to be addressed in future trials as nearly 25–30 % of patients present with distant metastases at some time point during the follow-up period.

1   Case Presentation

A 44-year-old male who has 20 pack/year smoking history with no significant past medical history presented with a painful mass in his right upper neck, which had gradually enlarged for nearly 8 months. He had no problems with dysphagia, swallowing, chewing, phonation as well as any chest pain, palpitations, or dyspnea.

His physical examination and rhinoscopy revealed normal ear and nasal findings. He had no dental problem. There were no lesions of the gingiva, buccal mucosa, floor of mouth, oral tongue, base of tongue, hard palate, soft palate, tonsillar fossa, or posterior oropharyngeal wall by visualization or palpation. There was an approximately 2 cm hardly mobile painful node in the left upper level II–III area and was no other palpable adenopathy on his left neck. Examinations of cranial nerves II–XII are grossly normal. On endoscopic examination, there was no evidence of disease in the oropharynx, larynx, and hypopharynx, and vocal cords were mobile, but mucosal surfaces were irregular on the left posterior wall of nasopharynx, which was randomly biopsied for two times with no evidence of malignancy.

On MRI and PET-CT, multiple hypermetabolic lymph nodes on left levels IIA, IIB, and III, greatest of which was measured 30×21 mm, were defined, but primary tumor origin could not be determined (Fig. 11.1).

A biopsy was performed from these lymph nodes confirming the metastatic carcinoma of squamous cell type.

He was staged as N2bM0 MCCUP.

2   Evidence-Based Treatment Approaches

Treatment plans are mainly tailored by the involved lymph node site and its association with probable primaries (Table 11.1), stage of neck (Table 11.2), surgical margin and extranodal extension (ECE) status, and presence/absence of residual disease. Neck dissection (ND) is the preferentially recommended treatment option for N1 patients with SCC histology, RT being an alternative Category 2B. RT is also

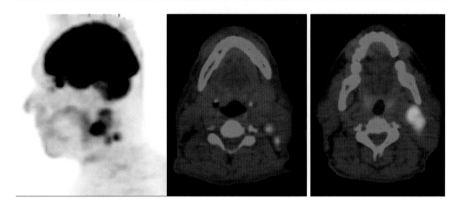

Fig. 11.1 Multiple hypermetabolic lymph nodes on left levels IIA, IIB, and III

Table 11.1 Nomenclature of neck lymph node regions and their relation with possible primary tumor sites

Level	Involved nodes	Possible primaries
1A	Submental	Lower lip, anterior tongue, floor of mouth
1B	Submandibular	Anterior alveolar mandibular ridge
		Oral cavity, anterior nasal cavity, submandibular glands
2A-B	Jugulodigastric/ upper jugular	Oral cavity, nasal cavity, nasopharynx, oropharynx,
		Hypopharynx, larynx, major salivary glands
		Oropharynx, nasopharynx
3	Middle jugular	Oropharynx, nasopharynx, oral cavity,
		Larynx, hypopharynx
4	Lower jugular	Larynx, hypopharynx, thyroid
		Cervical esophagus
5A-B	Posterior triangle	Nasopharynx, oropharynx, subglottic larynx,
		Apex of pyriform sinus, thyroid, cervical esophagus
6	Anterior compartment	Glottic and subglottic larynx, apex of pyriform sinus, thyroid, cervical esophagus
Retropharyngeal	Medial, lateral retropharyngeal	Nasopharynx, oropharynx, soft palate, hypopharynx

indicated in medically unfit patients or in technically unresectable N1 disease. In surgically treated patients, adjuvant treatment indications depend on the status of gross residue, surgical margins, ECE, and pathological nodal involvement. For N1 and ECE (−) patients, both observation and RT are options. For N2-3 and ECE (−) cases, RT or CRT (Category 2B) may be alternatives. If ECE (+), CRT is the treatment of choice (Category 1), but RT may be an option for cases unsuitable for chemotherapy. If gross residue left or surgical margins are positive, re-resection and/or CRT should be performed. In any patient planned to receive RT or CRT at upfront/adjuvant settings, it is mandatory to consider the tumor size, involved nodal

Table 11.2 Nodal staging for MCCUP (AJCC 7th edition)

Nodal disease	Nodal characteristics
N1	Metastasis in a single ipsilateral lymph node, 3 cm or less in greatest dimension
N2a	Metastasis in single ipsilateral lymph node more than 3 cm but not more than 6 cm in greatest dimension
N2b	Metastasis in multiple ipsilateral lymph nodes, none more than 6 cm in greatest dimension
N2c	Metastasis in bilateral or contralateral lymph nodes, none more than 6 cm in greatest dimension
N3	Metastasis in a lymph node more than 6 cm in greatest dimension

Abbreviations: AJCC American Joint Committee on Cancer, *MCCUP* Metastatic cervical cancer of unknown primary, *N* nodal stage

station(s), and HPV and EBV status for the design of RT field. Salvage ND is indicated in clinical or metabolic evidence of residual disease following RT or CRT.

CRT is the preferred upfront treatment option for all medically fit patients with N2–3 disease (Category 2B). Induction chemotherapy (Category 3) followed by RT or CRT is alternative recommendation for such patients. Salvage ND should be considered in patients with incomplete response.

In N1 and early N2A disease, either ND or RT alone provides excellent regional control rates. For ECE (−) N1-2a disease, neck recurrence rates following either modality ranges from 0 to 15 % [1, 2]. In adequately dissected ECE (−) cases, postoperative RT is not necessary as does not increase local control rates or survival [1, 3]. In ECE (+) patients, postoperative concurrent CRT is mandatory to increase local control rates [1].

In patients with advanced neck disease (N2b-N3), combined modality treatment with postoperative CRT or definitive CRT followed by planned ND for residual, unresponsive, or progressive tumors is the standard treatment approach with the best neck control and survival outcomes. In a series of 224 patients treated with RT alone, Grau et al. reported 5-year neck control and overall survival rates of 50 and 37 %, respectively [4]. In two recent smaller series with 40 and 60 patients, Aslani et al. [5] and Lu et al. [6] reported encouraging 5-year local control (76.3 and 65.3 %) and overall survival (77.8 and 68.5 %) rates, which may be associated with significant improvements in diagnostics and RT techniques. As a reflection of site specific data from advanced HNC which suggest significantly better locoregional control and survival rates with CRT than RT alone, it is rational to anticipate similar outcomes for MCCUP patients [7–9]. In series of definitive concurrent CRT or postoperative CRT, the 2- to 5-year rates of 89–100 % neck control and 74–92 % overall survival are excellent [10].

A summary of results of RT and CRT series of MCCUP are summarized in Table 11.3.

Although extensive-field RT including the bilateral neck and potentially involved mucosal sites is the widely practiced RT option, the question whether the irradiation

Table 11.3 Outcomes of patients with MCCUP following RT or CRT

	Outcome
Neck control[a]	
N1-2a	90–100 %
N2b-c	80 %
N3	50–60 %
Distant metastasis	
N1-2a	<10 %
N2b-c	15 %
N3	25 %
5-y overall survival	40–60 %
Emergence of primary[b]	
Median time	21 months
2-y	<10 %
5-y	15 %
10-y	20 %

Abbreviations: CRT chemoradiotherapy, *MCCUP* metastatic cervical cancer of unknown primary, *N* nodal stage, *RT* radiotherapy, *y* year
[a]Decreases with unilateral irradiation
[b]Decreases with irradiation of mucosal sites

be uni- or bilateral neck and whether potential mucosal sites be irradiated has not answered yet. Data from two literature reviews favor bilateral neck irradiation and inclusion of mucosal sites over unilateral neck irradiation alone [10, 11], but care must be given as different studies may have suffer from biases of inclusion of patients with poor overall health status or heavy/inoperable necks in unilateral neck irradiation group.

RT technique of choice is another question. However, a recent study by Ligey et al. demonstrated that use of 3D-RT or IMRT were associated with significantly superior regional control ($p=0.026$) and survival outcomes ($p=0.029$) compared to 2D-RT [12]. Based on the available data on specific HNC sites, IMRT has the similar potential to offer lesser acute and late toxicity rates for MCCUP patients, especially for cases in whom bilateral neck and/or mucosal sites are planned to be irradiated [13, 14]. Therefore, we recommend the use of 3D-RT as minimum standard, preferably IMRT where available.

Primary tumor emergence at mucosal sites is generally in the range of 0–12 % [15], increasing by time and decreasing with involvement of mucosal sites in the RT portal (Table 11.3). In series of Wallace et al., mucosal control rates for neck only and selective mucosal irradiation were 92 and 100 %, respectively [16]. Because majority of unknown primaries emerge at tonsils and base of tongue, the authors included nasopharynx and oropharynx in their selective radiation portal and included larynx and hypopharynx only in cases with level 3 nodal involvements. On the other hand, as their incidence rates are similar, it is rather difficult to discriminate true mucosal emergence of MCCUP from second primaries of head and neck area [17].

3   Target Volume Determination and Delineation Guidelines

Gross Tumor Volume (GTV)

GTV should encompass the any grossly involved lymph node(s), namely, >1 cm on shortest diameter with a necrotic center or metabolically active on PET scans, and with any apparent soft tissue extensions. All data from clinical and endoscopic examination, CT, MRI, and/or PET-CT should be comprehensively used for accurate GTV definition. Co-registered images may provide higher chance for correct delineation of GTV.

Clinical Target Volume (CTV)

Based on the risk definitions, 3 CTV volumes need to be defined:

- *CTV1:* For definitive RT/CRT or postsurgical patients with positive margins, CTV1 corresponds to GTV plus a margin of ≥5 mm at all directions, which may be reduced to as low as 1 mm in close proximity to critical structures. In postsurgical setting with soft tissue invasion or ECE (+), CTV1 is the surgical bed with a margin of ≥5 mm at all directions and represents for high-risk CTV1. In the absence of adverse factors, CTV1 is the surgical bed with a margin of ≥5 mm around and represents for intermediate risk CTV1.
- *CTV2:* It represents the high-risk region for subclinical disease including microscopic disease and potential routes of spread for likely primary and nodal disease. Potential primary regions should include the entire nasopharynx, base of tongue, ipsilateral tonsillar fossae, pyriform sinus, and highly suspected regions depending on the location and laterality of involved lymph node(s). For definitive RT/CRT or postsurgical patients with positive margins, CTV2 corresponds to soft tissues and nodal regions adjacent to CTV1. For soft tissue component, 0.5- to 1-cm margin around and for nodal component 2–3 cm from CTV1 nodal basins should be included in CTV2. In postoperative setting, CTV2 includes elective nodal regions and potential primary regions for both high- and intermediate-risk IMRT, as defined above.
- *CTV3:* Lower-risk elective nodal regions such as bilateral low anterior neck or contralateral neck in cases with unilateral lymph node involvement form the CTV3.

Planning Target Volume (PTV)

PTV is formed by additional margin around the CTVs to compensate for the intra- and/or inter-fraction variability, uncertainties of treatment setup, and internal organ motion. It is better for institutions to define their own PTV margin, which may

Table 11.4 Suggested lymph node levels to be included in radiotherapy portal according to suspected primary site

Suspected primary	N1-2a	N2b-3
Nasopharynx	1, 2, 3, 4, and RPN	2 3, 4, 5, and RPN
Oral cavity	1, 2, and 3 (4 if anterior tongue suspected)	1, 2, 3, 4, and 5
Oropharynx	2, 3, and 4 (RPN if posterior PWT suspected)	1, 2, 3, 4, 5, and RPN
Hypopharynx	2, 3, and 4	1, 2, 3, 4, 5, and RPN
Larynx	2, 3, and 4	2, 3, 4, and 5

Abbreviations: PWT posterior pharyngeal wall tumor, RPN retropharyngeal nodes

highly differ between RT centers. In general, a minimum of 5 mm at all directions is used to define each PTV. However, as it is critical to consider organs at risk, PTV margins can be reduced as needed. Respective PTV1, PTV2, and PTV3 are created by adding abovementioned margins to CTV1, CTV2, and CTV3.

Any MCCUP or primary HNC almost never involve all lymph node regions (level 1a to 6).

It should be kept in mind that the risk of ECE increases with size. Almost >50 % of lymph nodes between 1 and 3 cm are ECE (+), which increases to >75 % in tumors >3 cm [18–22].

Probable primary tumor sites according to involved lymph node station(s) are summarized in Table 11.1.

In addition to primary involved nodal basins, the probable intermediate risk or elective nodes to be involved in typical IMRT portal according to suspected primary sites should be defined as described in Table 11.4.

If bilateral node stations are involved, tumors of midline structures such as nasopharynx, hypopharynx, hard or soft palate, floor of mouth, and supraglottic larynx should specifically be remembered.

If exclusive level IV involvement is present, probable tumor site should highly be suspected below the clavicles.

Representative target volumes for MCCUP case presented here are shown in Fig. 11.2.

Level Definition Tips

Level IB (submandibular) is separated from level IIA by the submandibular gland and jugular vein interface, level II (subdigastric-jugulodigastric) follows the jugular vein to the jugular fossae, hyoid bone and upper border of cricoid cartilage separates level II from III (midjugular), level IV (low jugular and supraclavicular) lays between lower border of cricoids cartilage and clavicle, and level V (posterior cervical) nodes are located behind posterior edge of sternocleidomastoid muscle.

Fig. 11.2 Representative target volumes for metastatic cervical cancer of unknown primary case presented here (**a**, **b**)

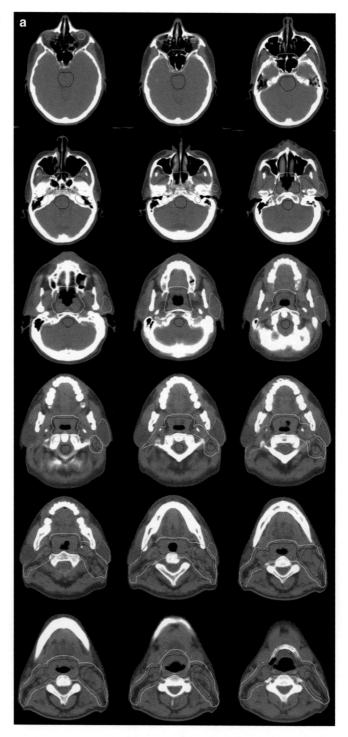

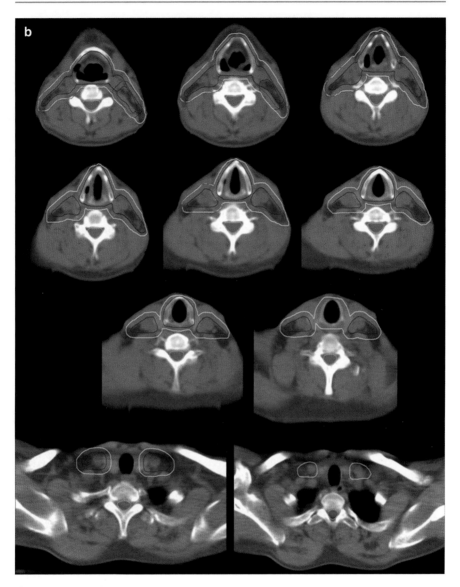

Fig. 11.2 (continued)

Case Contouring (Fig. 11.2)

- Check coverage of nasopharynx
- Check coverage of base of tongue
- Check coverage of uni- or bilateral tonsils

- Check coverage of pyriform sinus
- Check coverage of additional head and neck structures based on nodal involvement
- Check coverage of the midline structures in case of bilateral nodal involvement

4   Treatment Planning

- *Guidelines for Radiotherapy Doses:* To minimize dose to the critical structures, particularly the parotid glands, IMRT (preferred) or 3D-RT is recommended. This is critical especially when oropharyngeal structures are included in radiation portal. Dose distribution of PTV_{70}, $PTV_{59.4}$, and PTV_{54} Gy and related dose-volume histogram for the case presented here are demonstrated in Figs. 11.3 and 11.4, respectively. Typical recommended doses of RT for definitive RT/CRT and postoperative settings are described in Table 11.5.

Definitive Radiotherapy

- *High-Risk PTV*: Includes involved lymph nodes and possible local subclinical infiltration at the high-risk level lymph node(s). A total of 66 Gy (2.2 Gy/fr) or 70 Gy (2 Gy/fr or 2.12 Gy/fr if dose-painting IMRT or simultaneous integrated boost IMRT used. If the planned dose is >70 Gy, in an effort to minimize the risk of toxicity, some authors recommend use of slightly decreased daily doses (e.g. <2 Gy) at least during some part of treatment.
- *Mucosal Sites*: Depending on the field size, putative mucosal sites should receive 50–66 Gy (2 Gy/fr) with standard 3D-RT or sequentially planned IMRT. For highly suspicious mucosal sites, 60–66 Gy should be considered. If dose-painting IMRT or simultaneous integrated boost IMRT is utilized, doses of 54–66 Gy (1.63–2 Gy/fr in 33 fractions) are recommended as indicated.
- *Low-Intermediate Risk PTV*: All suspected sites of subclinical spread including the nasopharynx, base of tongue, tonsils, pyriform sinus, and bilateral neck nodes (levels I–V):
  - In cases of 3D-RT or sequentially planned IMRT: 44–50 Gy in 2 Gy daily fractions
  - If IMRT is dose painting or simultaneous integrated boost: 54–63 Gy in 1.6–1.8 Gy daily fractions

Definitive Concurrent Chemoradiotherapy

- *High-Risk PTV*: Typical dose is 70 Gy (2 Gy/fr) for 3D-RT or dose painting IMRT/simultaneous integrated boost (2.12 Gy/fr). Doses beyond 70 Gy is not recommended with concurrent CRT.

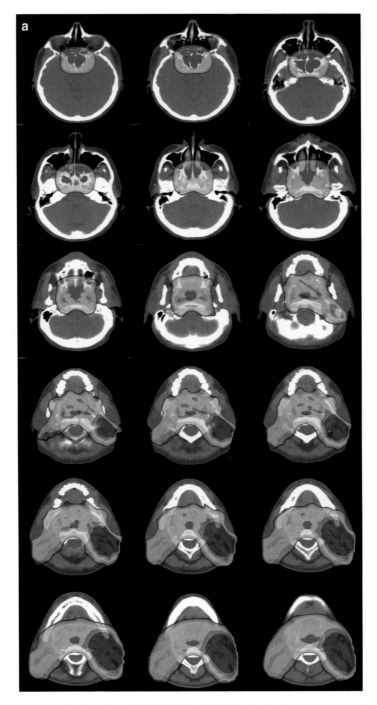

Fig. 11.3 Dose distribution of PTV70, PTV59.4, and PTV 54 Gy for the case presented here (**a**, **b**)

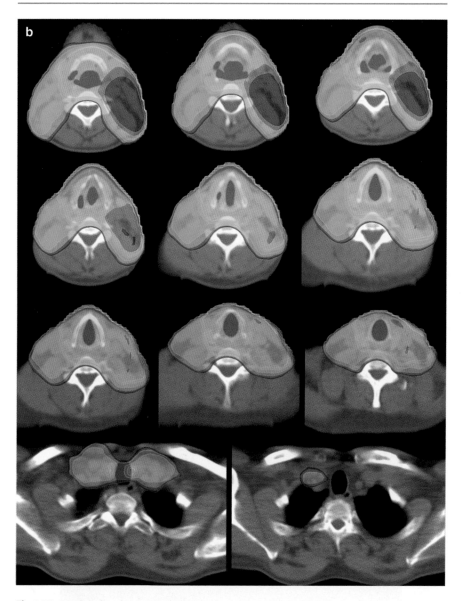

Fig. 11.3 (continued)

- *Mucosal Sites:* Depending on the field size, putative mucosal sites should receive 50–66 Gy (2 Gy/fr) with standard 3D-RT or sequentially planned IMRT. For highly suspicious mucosal sites, 60–66 Gy should be considered. If dose-painting IMRT or simultaneous integrated boost IMRT is utilized, doses of 54–66 Gy (1.63–2 Gy/fr in 33 fractions) are recommended as indicated.

Table 11.5 Recommendations for RT doses and fractionation for target volumes with standard or simultaneous integrated boost IMRT

Treatment type	PTV1	PTV2	PTV3
Definitive RT	66–70 Gy (2–2.12 Gy/fr)	59.4–66 Gy (1.8–2 Gy/fr)	46–54 Gy (1.63–2 Gy)
Definitive CRT	66–70 Gy (2–2.12 Gy/fr)	59.4–66 Gy (1.8–2 Gy/fr)	46–54 Gy (1.63–2 Gy)
Postoperative RT			
Risk factors (+)	66–70 Gy (2–2.12 Gy/fr)	59.4–66 Gy (1.8–2 Gy/fr)	46–54 Gy (1.63–2 Gy)
Risk factors (−)	60–66 Gy (2–2.12 Gy/fr)	54–63 Gy (1.8–1.9 Gy/fr)	46–54 Gy (1.63–2 Gy)
Postoperative CRT			
Risk factors (+)	66–70 Gy (2–2.12 Gy/fr)	59.4–66 Gy (1.8–2 Gy/fr)	46-54 Gy (1.63–2 Gy)
Risk factors (−)	60–66 Gy (2–2.12 Gy/fr)	54–63 Gy (1.8–1.9 Gy/fr)	46–54 Gy (1.63–2 Gy)

Abbreviations: *CRT* chemoradiotherapy, *IMRT* intensity-modulated radiation therapy, *PTV* Planning target volume, *RT* radiotherapy

- *Low-Intermediate-Risk PTV:* All suspected sites of subclinical spread including the nasopharynx, base of tongue, tonsils, pyriform sinus, and bilateral neck nodes (levels I–V)
  - In cases of 3D-RT or sequentially planned IMRT: 44–50 Gy in 2 Gy daily fractions
  - If IMRT is dose painting or simultaneous integrated boost: 54–63 Gy in 1.6–1.8 Gy daily fractions

Postoperative Radiotherapy

- Radiotherapy should preferentially commence on ≤6 weeks of postoperative period.
- *High-Risk PTV:* Includes the surgical field with adverse factors such as ECE (+) and/or close/positive surgical margins. Typical dose is 59.4–66 Gy (1.8–2 Gy/fr) for patients with ECE (+) and/or close surgical margins with concurrent chemotherapy. For patients with positive surgical margins, a dose of 70 Gy (2 Gy/fr) is recommended for 3D-RT or standard IMRT. If dose-painting IMRT or simultaneous integrated boost IMRT is used, then the dose is 70 Gy in 2.12 Gy daily fractions.
- *Mucosal Sites:* Depending on the field size, putative mucosal sites should receive 50–66 Gy (2 Gy/fr) with standard 3D-RT or sequentially planned IMRT. For highly suspicious mucosal sites, 60–66 Gy should be considered. If dose-painting

IMRT or simultaneous integrated boost IMRT is utilized, doses of 54–66 Gy (1.63–2 Gy/fr in 33 fractions) are recommended as indicated.

- *Low-Intermediate-Risk PTV:* All suspected sites of subclinical spread including the nasopharynx, base of tongue, tonsils, pyriform sinus, and bilateral neck nodes (levels I–V)
  - In cases of 3D-RT or sequentially planned IMRT: 44–50 Gy in 2 Gy daily fractions
  - If IMRT is dose painting or simultaneous integrated boost: 54–63 Gy in 1.6–1.8 Gy daily fractions

Postoperative Chemoradiotherapy

- Radiotherapy should preferentially commence on ≤6 weeks of postoperative period.
- Single-agent cisplatin at 100 mg/m^2 every 3 weeks is recommended concurrently with RT. Weekly use of cisplatin may be an alternative for patients anticipated to hardly tolerate or intolerate standard cisplatin protocol.
- *High-Risk PTV:* Includes the surgical field with adverse factors such as ECE (+) and/or close/positive surgical margins. Typical dose is 59.4–66 Gy (1.8–2 Gy/fr) for patients with ECE (+) and/or close surgical margins. For patients with positive surgical margins, a dose of 70 Gy (2 Gy/fr) is recommended for 3D-RT or standard IMRT. If dose-painting IMRT or simultaneous integrated boost IMRT is used, then the dose is 70 Gy in 2.12 Gy daily fractions.
- *Mucosal Sites:* Depending on the field size, putative mucosal sites should receive 50–66 Gy (2 Gy/fr) with standard 3D-RT or sequentially planned IMRT. For highly suspicious mucosal sites, 60–66 Gy should be considered. If dose-painting IMRT or simultaneous integrated boost IMRT is utilized, doses of 54–66 Gy (1.63–2 Gy/fr in 33 fractions) are recommended as indicated.
- *Low-Intermediate-Risk PTV:* All suspected sites of subclinical spread including the nasopharynx, base of tongue, tonsils, pyriform sinus, and bilateral neck nodes (levels I–V)
  - In cases of 3D-RT or sequentially planned IMRT: 44–50 Gy in 2 Gy daily fractions
  - If IMRT is dose painting or simultaneous integrated boost: 54–63 Gy in 1.6–1.8 Gy daily fractions
- *Guidelines for Normal Tissue Constraints:* Normal tissue dose constraints detailed below should strictly be obeyed to prevent debilitating late toxicities. Dose-volume histogram of critical organ doses for the present representative patient is demonstrated in Fig. 11.4:
  - Parotid glands: mean dose (D_{mean}) of ≤26 Gy or less *(should be achieved in at least one gland)* or at least 20 cc of the combined volume of both glands should receive <20 Gy or at least 50 % of one parotid gland should receive <30 Gy.). Brain stem: maximum dose (D_{max}) ≤54 Gy

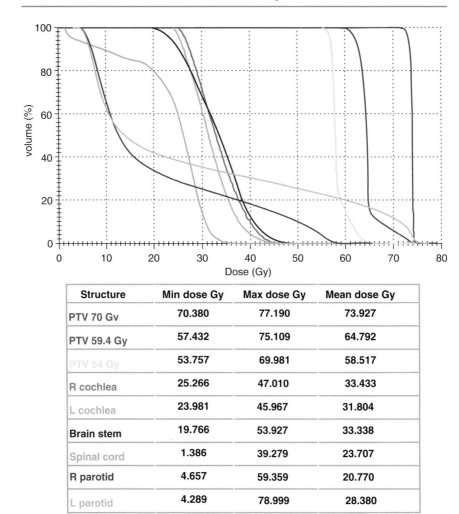

Structure	Min dose Gy	Max dose Gy	Mean dose Gy
PTV 70 Gv	70.380	77.190	73.927
PTV 59.4 Gy	57.432	75.109	64.792
PTV 54 Gy	53.757	69.981	58.517
R cochlea	25.266	47.010	33.433
L cochlea	23.981	45.967	31.804
Brain stem	19.766	53.927	33.338
Spinal cord	1.386	39.279	23.707
R parotid	4.657	59.359	20.770
L parotid	4.289	78.999	28.380

Fig. 11.4 Dose-volume histogram of prescribed target volume doses and critical organs at risk

- Spinal cord: $D_{max} \leq 45$ Gy oral cavity: $D_{mean} <30$ to 35 Gy
- Brain: $D_{max} \leq 50$ Gy and any large volume of brain should receive <30 Gy
- Optic nerve, optic chiasm: $D_{max} <54$ Gy
- Lens: D_{max} is 10 Gy, and <5Gy if achievable
- Mandible: $D_{max} <69$ Gy (hot spots >70Gy should be kept out of the mandible).
- Cochlea: no more than 5 % receives ≥ 55 Gy
- Glottic Larynx: $D_{mean} <36$–45 Gy, if not suspected as potential primary

Table 11.6 IMRT plan assessment specifications

PTV	No variation	Minor variation
PTV_{70}	1. 95 % of any PTV_{70} is at or above 70 Gy	1. 95 % of PTV_{70} is at or above 70 Gy
	2. 99 % of PTV_{70} is at or above 65.1 Gy	2. 97 % of PTV_{70} is at or above 65.1 Gy
	3. No more than 20 % of PTV_{70} is at or above 77 Gy	3. No more than 40 % of PTV_{70} is at or above 77 Gy
	4. No more than 5 % of PTV_{70} is at or above 80 Gy	4. No more than 20 % of PTV_{70} is at or above 80 Gy
	5. Mean dose $\leq$74 Gy	5. Mean dose $\leq$76 Gy
PTV_{63} (if applicable)	1. 95 % of any PTV_{63} is at or above 63 Gy	1. 95 % of any PTV_{63} is at or above 58.6 Gy
	2. 99 % of PTV_{63} is at or above 58.6 Gy	2. No more than 40 % of PTV_{63} is at or above 77 Gy
	3. No more than 20 % of PTV_{63} is at or above 77 Gy	3. No more than 20 % of PTV_{63} is at or above 80 Gy
	4. No more than 5 % of PTV_{63} is at or above 80 Gy	
$PTV_{59.4}$	1. 95 % of any $PTV_{59.4}$ is at or above 59.4 Gy	1. 95 % of $PTV_{59.4}$ is at or above 55.2 Gy
	2. 99 % of $PTV_{59.4}$ is at or above 55.2 Gy	2. No more than 40 % of $PTV_{59.4}$ is at or above 77 Gy
	3. No more than 20 % of $PTV_{59.4}$ is at or above 77 Gy	3. No more than 20 % of $PTV_{59.4}$ is at or above 80 Gy
	4. No more than 5 % of $PTV_{59.4}$ is at or above 80 Gy	
PTV_{54} (if applicable)	1. 95 % of any PTV_{54} is at/or above 54 Gy	1. 95 % of PTV_{54} is at or above 50.2 Gy
	2. 99 % of PTV_{54} is at or above 50.2 Gy	2. No more than 40 % of PTV_{54} is at or above 65.3 Gy
	3. No more than 20 % of PTV_{54} is at or above 65.3 Gy	3. No more than 20 % of PTV_{54} is at or above 68.3 Gy
	4. No more than 5 % of PTV_{54} is at or above 68.3 Gy	

Abbreviations: IMRT intensity-modulated radiation therapy, *PTV* planning target volume (subscript denotes for prescribed dose)

- *Treatment Planning AssessmentStep 1:* Check whether the targets are adequately covered. As a common example recommended assessment specifications in Table 11.6 are given for typical dose prescriptions of PTV1 (PTV_{70}), PTV2 ($PTV_{59.4}$), and PTV3 (PTV_{54}). However, as various scenarios of patient presentation are possible (definitive RT, definitive CRT, postoperative RT with/without adverse factors, and postoperative CRT with/without adverse factors), all dose coverage values presented in percentages should also be used for any prescribed dose levels. All plans

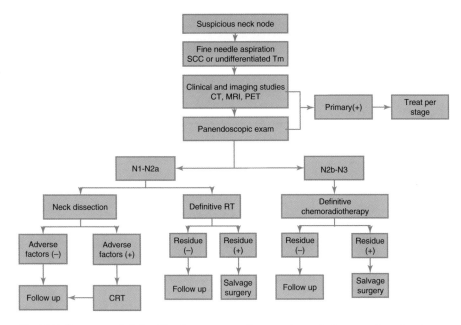

Fig. 11.5 Recommended algorithm for treatment of metastatic cervical cancer of occult primary

should be normalized to at least 95 % of the volumes of PTV1, PTV2, and PTV3 are covered by the 100 % of respectively prescribed isodose surfaces and 99 % of each PTV should be covered by 93 % of prescribed doses.
– Minor deviations are acceptable only for few assessment points where critical organ tolerance doses limit achieve excellent target coverage.
   – *Step 2:* Presence of a large hot spot should be carefully checked and should not be permitted for more than 20 % of PTV1 (e.g. 70 Gy) to receive $\geq$110 % and no more than 5 % of PTV1 to receive $\geq$%115 of prescribed dose, respectively.
   – *Step 3:* Normal tissue constraints should carefully be checked.
   – *Step 4:* Plan should be checked slide by slide via examining the isodose distribution to prevent the hot and cold spots not to exist on critical organs.
   – *Step 5:* Hot spots should be restricted to the GTV with being sure that the hot spot does not coincide on any nerve in the CTV.
• *Case Plan:* The patient with locally advanced MCCUP presented here was treated with concurrent CRT (cisplatin 100 mg/m^2, every 21 days) utilizing SIB-IMRT technique. As demonstrated in Figs. 11.2, 11.3 and 11.4, the prescribed doses for PTV1, PTV2, and PTV3 were 70, 59.4, and 54 Gy in 33 fractions, respectively.
• *Treatment Algorithm and Patient Follow-Up:* Recommended evidence-based treatment options and patient follow-up after treatment for MCCUP patients are as depicted in Figs. 11.5 and 11.6, respectively.

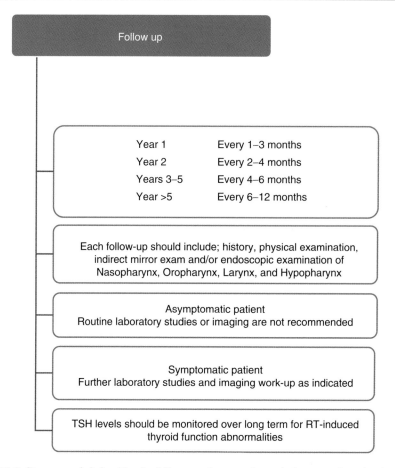

Fig. 11.6 Recommended algorithm for follow-up of metastatic cervical cancer of occult primary

References

1. Strojan P, Ferlito A, Langendijk JA et al (2013) Contemporary management of lymph node metastases from an unknown primary to the neck: II. a review of therapeutic options. Head Neck 35(2):286–293
2. Colletier PJ, Garden AS, Morrison WH et al (1998) Postoperative radiation for squamous cell carcinoma metastatic to cervical lymph nodes from an unknown primary site: outcomes and patterns of failure. Head Neck 20:674–681
3. Rodrigo JP, Maseda E, Maldonado M et al (2004) Efficacy of postoperative radiation therapy for squamous cell carcinoma of the head and neck: results of a prospective randomised clinical trial. Acta Otorrinolaringol Esp 55:415–419
4. Grau C, Johansen LV, Jakobsen J et al (2000) Cervical lymph node metastases from unknown primary tumours. Results from a national survey by the Danish Society for Head and Neck Oncology. Radiother Oncol 55(2):121–129

5. Aslani M, Sultanem K, Voung T et al (2007) Metastatic carcinoma to the cervical nodes from an unknown head and neck primary site: Is there a need for neck dissection? Head Neck 29(6):585–590
6. Lu X, Hu C, Ji Q et al (2009) Squamous cell carcinoma metastatic to cervical lymph nodes from an unknown primary site: the impact of radiotherapy. Tumori 95(2):185–190
7. Forastiere AA, Zhang Q, Weber RS et al (2013) Long-term results of RTOG 91–11: a comparison of three nonsurgical treatment strategies to preserve the larynx in patients with locally advanced larynx cancer. J Clin Oncol 31:845–852
8. Lefebvre JL, Andry G, Chevalier D et al (2012) Laryngeal preservation with induction chemotherapy for hypopharyngeal squamous cell carcinoma: 10-year results of EORTC trial 24891. Ann Oncol 23:2708–2714
9. Blanchard P, Baujat B, Holostenco V, MACH-CH Collaborative group et al (2011) Meta-analysis of chemotherapy in head and neck cancer (MACH-NC): a comprehensive analysis by tumour site. Radiother Oncol 100(1):33–40
10. Nieder C, Gregoire V, Ang KK (2001) Cervical lymph node metastases from occult squamous cell carcinoma: cut down a tree to get an apple? Int J Radiat Oncol Biol Phys 50:727–733
11. Jereczek–Fossa BA, Jassem J, Orecchia R (2004) Cervical lymph node metastases of squamous cell carcinoma of unknown primary. Cancer Treat Rev 30:153–164
12. Ligey A, Gentil J, Créhange G et al (2009) Impact of target volumes and radiation technique on loco-regional control and survival for patients with unilateral cervical lymph node metastases from an unknown primary. Radiother Oncol 93(3):483–487
13. Chajon E, Lafond C, Louvel G et al (2013) Salivary gland-sparing other than parotid-sparing in definitive head-and-neck intensity-modulated radiotherapy does not seem to jeopardize local control. Radiat Oncol 8(1):132
14. O'Sullivan B, Rumble RB, Warde P (2012) Intensity-modulated radiotherapy in the treatment of head and neck cancer. Clin Oncol (R Coll Radiol) 24(7):474–487
15. Strojan P, Anicin A (1998) Combined surgery and postoperative radiotherapy for cervical lymph node metastases from an unknown primary tumour. Radiother Oncol 49(1):33–40
16. Wallace A, Richards GM, Harari PM et al (2011) Head and neck squamous cell carcinoma from an unknown primary site. Am J Otolaryngol 32(4):286–290
17. Harper CS, Mendenhall WM, Parsons JT et al (1990) Cancer in neck nodes with unknown primary site: role of mucosal radiotherapy. Head Neck 12:463–469
18. Johnson JT, Barnes EL, Myers EN et al (1981) The extracapsular spread of tumors in cervical node metastasis. Arch Otolaryngol 107(12):725–729
19. Snow GB, Annyas AA, van Slooten EA et al (1982) Prognostic factors of neck node metastasis. Clin Otolaryngol Allied Sci 7(3):185–192
20. Snyderman NL, Johnson JT, Schramm VL Jr et al (1985) Extracapsular spread of carcinoma in cervical lymph nodes. Impact upon survival in patients with carcinoma of the supraglottic larynx. Cancer 56(7):1597–1599
21. Hirabayashi H, Koshii K, Uno K et al (1991) Extracapsular spread of squamous cell carcinoma in neck lymph nodes: prognostic factor of laryngeal cancer. Laryngoscope 101(5):502–506
22. Lee N, Xia P, Quivey JM et al (2002) Intensity-modulated radiotherapy in the treatment of nasopharyngeal carcinoma: an update of the UCSF experience. Int J Radiat Oncol Biol Phys 53(1):12–22

Complications of Head and Neck Radiotherapy and Management

12

Murat Beyzadeoglu, Ferrat Dincoglan, and Omer Sager

Overview

Emerging technological advances in the field of radiation oncology allows for more refined treatments with improved delineation of target and critical structures by means of supplementary data from multimodality imaging and precise treatment delivery under image guidance. Understanding of the interactions of radiation with chemotherapeutics and biological response modifiers is improving as the relevant data accumulates and this contributes to understanding of normal tissue toxicities.

Radiation-related normal tissue toxicity may occur both during the course of radiation therapy and after treatment completion. The incidence of radiation morbidity may be dependent on the treatment technique, tumor volume and disease extent, the size of treatment field, time-dose-fractionation features, and patient-related factors including age, nutritional status, and comorbidities. However, the effect of these factors on early and late responding tissues may show diversity. A formidable challenge of radiation therapy is that there is no selectivity of radiation for a certain body site or tissue, which causes varying degrees of morbidity particularly in the presence of close proximity of critical organ-at-risk structures to the target volume. In this aspect, normal tissue tolerance limits are of utmost importance in designing radiotherapy plans for any cancer type. Although constituting a relatively small portion of the human body, head and neck region contains critical parts associated with basic vital physiological functions including respiration, nutrition, and expression which emphasize the significance of radiation morbidity at the very outset. Since radiation dose essential for head and neck cancer eradication typically exceeds the normal tissue tolerance limits, vigilance is required to achieve optimal balance between treatment toxicity and cure.

M. Beyzadeoglu, MD (✉) • F. Dincoglan, MD • O. Sager, MD
Department of Radiation Oncology, Gulhane Military Medical School, Etlik, Ankara, Turkey
e-mail: mbeyzadeoglu@yahoo.com

© Springer International Publishing Switzerland 2015
M. Beyzadeoglu et al. (eds.), *Radiation Therapy for Head and Neck Cancers:
A Case-Based Review*, DOI 10.1007/978-3-319-10413-3_12

1 Introduction

Radiation sensitivity of tissues is determined by its precursor cells [1]. Cells vary in their inherent susceptibility to radiation. According to Bergonie and Tribondeau law, factors affecting tissue radiosensitivity include excessive less-differentiated cells in the tissue, abundant active mitotic cells, and the duration of active cell proliferation [1, 2]. Rapid cell turnover rate of the mucosal lining of upper respiratory and gastrointestinal tract makes it more susceptible to effects of radiation. Thus, the oral cavity with high mucosal turnover rate is prone to toxicity at high radiation exposure. Direct lethal and sublethal damage of the oral tissues along with immune system impairment may contribute to several acute and late complications including mucositis, xerostomia, pain, loss of taste, dysphagia and swallowing dysfunction, otitis externa and otitis media, periodontal disease and caries, soft tissue necrosis, mandibular osteoradionecrosis, temporomandibular joint dysfunction, trismus, fibrosis, endocrine dysfunctions, laryngeal edema, skin reactions, dehydration, dysgeusia, malnutrition, cataract formation, temporal lobe necrosis, myelitis, and second malignancies.

2 Mucositis

Radiation-induced basal cells loss of oral mucosal epithelium results in oral mucositis. Severity may be variable from mild discomfort to severe pain. Major patient-related risk factors include poor oral hygiene, periodontal caries, poor nutrition, tobacco, and alcohol use. Time-dose-fractionation features, tumor site, the use of concomitant chemotherapy, and surgical treatment are treatment-related risk factors. Mucositis is an exudative reaction which may progress from patchy to confluent mucositis. Typical symptoms include tenderness, erythema, edema, pain, and swallowing difficulties. A pseudomembrane, and a painful ulcerated surface resulting from membrane sloughing may occur. Onset of symptoms usually occurs 2 weeks after radiotherapy commencement and may persist up to 1 month after treatment completion or even longer particularly when concomitant chemotherapy is used (Fig. 12.1).

Minimizing the exposure of affected mucosa by tobacco, alcohol, or poorly fitting dentures should be considered in the management of mucositis. Optimizing the nutritional status of the patient and giving instructions for oral hygiene may aid in management. Saline and bicarbonate lavage may be used in the management of non-confluent mucositis. Topical xylocaine and other analgesics may be used to relieve oral discomfort. Treatment breaks should be avoided due to the accelerated repopulation features of the tumor.

Oral hygiene and mouth care are of utmost importance for decreasing the incidence and severity of oral complications. Patient education about the rationale for oral hygiene should be considered at the very outset. Effective oral hygiene maintenance is required throughout the treatment course to avoid complications. Frequent rinsing (four to six times daily) of the oral cavity with 0.9 % saline is common

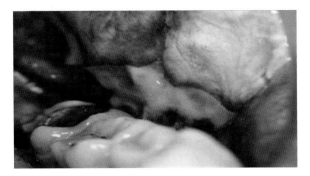

Fig. 12.1 Radiation-induced mucositis with incipient breakdown of the buccal mucosa (Reproduced with permission of Springer Science and Business Media)

practice in many centers. Avoiding the use of drying agents such as alcohol or glycerine-based products may be beneficial. Dental brushing with toothpaste, dental flossing, sodium bicarbonate rinses, and ice chips are useful in achieving bacterial dental plaque control. Cleaning of the oral cavity after meals is important. Reduced salivary function as a result of xerostomia may cause accumulation of food and debris, which requires more frequent hygiene.

Lip care products including petroleum-based oils and waxes may be used to avoid dryness of the lips.

Instruction of patients for routine follow-up with an expert dentist is crucial. A meticulous dental assessment several weeks before radiotherapy commencement is required to allow for adequate time interval for tissue healing if invasive oral procedures such as dental extraction are indicated. The potential risk of soft tissue necrosis and osteoradionecrosis may be reduced with this timely approach [3, 4].

Oral candidiasis is a frequent infection of the oropharynx in patients receiving radiotherapy to the head and neck region. This infection may aggravate mucositis since the yeast colonize the injured mucosa. Topical antifungals such as nystatin and clotrimazole may be used in the management of oral candidiasis. Systemic antifungals such as flucanozole and ketoconazole may also be used if necessary.

Mucosal healing usually occurs rapidly after completing radiation treatment.

3   Taste Changes

Atrophy and degeneration of taste buds may result as a consequence of oral cavity irradiation. Taste buds are susceptible to irradiation, and sensations of sweet, sour, salty, or bitter may be affected. Incidence of taste changes is dependent on radiation dose. Though recovery may be observed within a few months following treatment in some patients, persistent changes may also occur.

Patients should be instructed to chew foods longer to allow for more contact of foods with taste buds. Also, smelling the foods before eating may be recommended since taste and smelling senses are interlinked.

4   Xerostomia

Reduction in salivary flow as a result of salivary gland damage is a frequent complication of head and neck radiotherapy. Saliva is required for normal execution of oral
functions including swallowing, taste, and speech. So, permanent impairment of
salivary function may have several clinical consequences and may substantially
affect qualiy of life. As the salivary viscosity increases, lubrication of oral tissues is
impaired and buffering capacity is compromised with increased risk of dental caries
and progressive periodontal disease. Due to the patient's difficulty in maintaining
oral hygiene and mechanical cleansing, oral flora becomes more pathogenic and
plaque levels accumulate.

Unstimulated whole salivary flow rates under 0.1 mL/min are indicators of xerostomia. Significant reduction of salivary gland within the necrosis field causes xerostomia [5]. Typical symptoms and signs include dryness, fissures at lip commissures,
burning sensation of the tongue, a dorsal tongue surface atrophy, increased thirst,
and difficulty in wearing dentures (Fig. 12.2).

Xerostomia occurs as a result of inflammatory and degenerative effects of radiation on the salivary gland parenchyma. Salivary flow decreases within the first week
after radiotherapy commencement, and continual progressive decrease occurs during the course of treatment. The severity of hypofunction is dependent on the dose
of radiation and volume of glandular tissue within the radiotherapy field. Severe
radiotherapy-induced xerostomia with less than 25 % of the baseline salivary function may be avoided by sparing at least one parotid gland to a mean dose of <20 Gy
or by sparing both parotid glands to <25 Gy [6]. Nevertheless, keeping the parotid
mean doses as low as possible without compromising clinical target volume coverage is recommended since better function of the parotid glands may be achieved
with lower parotid mean doses [6].

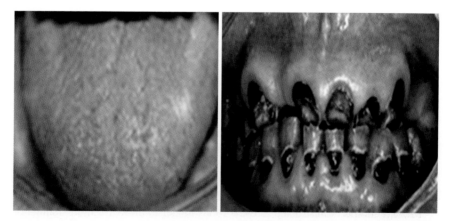

Fig. 12.2 Radiation-induced xerostomia and dental caries secondary to radiation therapy
(Reproduced with permission of Springer Science and Business Media)

Patients with xerostomia should maintain their oral hygiene to minimize the risk of oral lesion formation. Unless preventive measures are taken, periodontal disease may deteriorate and caries may become uncontrollable. Preventive strategies include plaque removal by toothbrushing and flossing; remineralization by the use of topical and/or systemic remineralizing solutions; rinsing with antimicrobials such as chlorhexidine, povidone iodine, etc.; and using sialogogues such as pilocarpine and bethanechol.

Surgical interventions may be used in the management of xerostomia [7–9]. Complementary methods such as acupuncture have been used for xerostomia prevention [10, 11].

Amifostine (WR-2721), which is a pro-drug dephosphorylated by plasma membrane alkaline phosphatase to the active metabolite of free thiol WR-1065, exerts its radioprotective action by scavenging free radicals produced by head and neck irradiation along with its detoxification effect used in chemotherapy-induced renal toxicity reduction. It is used as a radioprotective agent to reduce xerostomia in patients with head and neck cancers who are receiving radiotherapy [12–15].

Temporarily wetting the oral mucosa by saliva substitutes or artificial saliva preparations is a palliative cytoprotective strategy to relieve discomfort of patients with xerostomia.

Pilocarpine, a parasymppathomimetic agent, is used in the management of radiotherapy-induced xerostomia [16–18]. It may have a radioprotective effect on salivary glands if used during head and neck radiotherapy. Pilocarpine typically increases salivary flow within 30 min after ingestion. Continual use is required to achieve maximal benefit. Treatment is initiated at 5 mg orally, thrice daily, and dose is then titrated to achieve optimal balance between clinical response and side effects. Allowing a week between dose increments is recommended to confirm patient tolerance. Hyperhidrosis is a common adverse effect of pilocarpine.

5 Skin Toxicity

An overwhelming majority of patients receiving radiotherapy for head and neck cancers experience varying degrees of acute skin effects. Treatment-related factors include total dose, dose per fraction, type and energy of radiation, use of beam modifiers, the size of radiotherapy fields, and the use of concomitant therapeutic agents such as chemotherapeutics, radiosensitizers, monoclonal antibodies, etc. Patient-related risk factors include impaired nutritional status, fair complexion, history of extensive sun exposure, comorbid diseases such as diabetes mellitus, and collagen vascular diseases such as scleroderma and lupus.

Skin reactions range from mild erythema or dryness to dry or moist desquamation. Symptoms are usually temporary. Typical onset of symptoms occurs approximately 2 weeks after the commencement of radiotherapy and may persist up to 4 weeks after treatment completion (Fig. 12.3).

Management of skin toxicity includes adhering to principles of good wound care and maintaining a clean environment. Careful cleansing of the skin is warranted. Moisturizers (Acuophor or aloe vera gels) may be applied to areas of dry

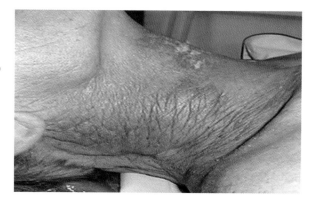

Fig. 12.3 Typical skin reaction after head and neck radiotherapy (Reproduced with permission of Springer Science and Business Media)

desquamation. Mechanical and chemical irritation of treated skin must be prevented by avoiding tight clothes, perfumes, etc. In the presence of moist desquamation, additional measures should be taken to avoid skin infections and consequential treatment breaks.

6 Osteoradionecrosis

Direct osteocytic damage or injury to the small vasculature of the haversian systems and the periosteum by irradiation may negatively affect the bone's capability to resist trauma and avoid infections. Pathologic fractures may occur since the compromised bone has lost its ability to repair itself. Pain, fistula, infection, and complete or partial sensational loss may occur.

Osteoradionecrosis typically involves the mandible in head and neck radiotherapy with varying incidences reported in retrospective series. The risk of osteoradionecrosis increases with trauma, oral infections, and intimate association of primary tumor with the bone. Osteoradionecrosis typically occurs within the first 3 years after diagnosis of head and neck cancer (Figs. 12.4 and 12.5).

Management of osteoradionecrosis includes the maintenance of meticulous oral hygiene, elimination of trauma, avoidance of removable dental prostheses when the denture bearing area is within the necrosis field, maintenance of adequate nutritional intake, and discontinuation of alcohol and tobacco consumption [19]. If attempts to preserve teeth are unsuccessful, postradiotherapy dental extractions should be performed cautiously due to the risk of initiating osteonecrosis. Topical or systemic antibiotics may be used in the presence of infection. Analgesics may be indicated for pain management. Local resection of loose bony spicules may be possible. Hyperbaric oxygen treatment may be recommended if conservative treatment has failed and the patient suffers from increasing pain. It may result inconsiderable pain relief through increased oxygenation of irradiated tissue, enhanced angiogenesis, increased osteoblast repopulation, and fibroblast function.

Surgical resection of the irradiated mandible may be indicated in severe cases of osteoradionecrosis. Reconstruction of the mandible may be considered to achieve continuity for esthetics and functionality. A multidisciplinary approach is warranted in the management of these patients.

Fig. 12.4 Skin breakdown and osteoradionecrosis of the mandibular angle and ascending ramus after radiotherapy for a parotid gland tumor (Reproduced with permission of Springer Science and Business Media)

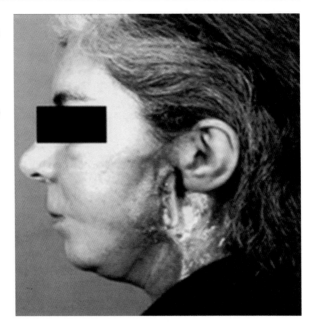

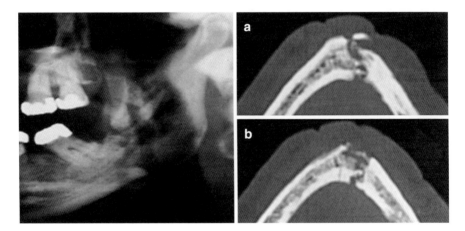

Fig. 12.5 Radiological aspects of osteoradionecrosis. Mixed radio-opaque radiolucent lesion, with the radiolucent areas representing bone destruction and axial CT of the mandible with osteo-radionecrosis showing (**a**) small sequestra of bone (**b**) symphysis pathological fracture (Reproduced with permission of Springer Science and Business Media)

7   Soft Tissue Necrosis

Necrosis of the soft tissue is a rare complication and mostly occurs due to an ill-fitting prosthesis or when a very highly focused dose of radiation is delivered such as with an interstitial implant [20]. Considering that the mucosa and gingiva continue to change up to several months after irradiation, it is preferable to avoid making a new prosthesis for at least 3 months after radiotherapy completion. Usage of any ill-fitting prosthesis should be avoided since it would serve as a continued source of irritation.

If there is no underlying recurrent tumor, conservative management with oral hygiene, antibiotics, and rarely hyperbaric oxygen may be adequate for tissue healing [20].

8   Fibrosis

Subcutaneous fibrosis may occur as a severe complication in the neck, particularly in the presence of a neck dissection. Submental edema (turkey waddle) may develop which typically subsides after several months [20]. Exercise may prevent the formation of contractures.

9   Trismus

Trismus typically results from formation of fibrosis around the masticatory muscles and the temporomandibular joint. Radiation alone may cause trismus; however, it is more commonly seen when radiation is delivered in the postoperative setting. Stretching exercises may be useful in the management of trismus [20].

10   Endocrine Dysfunction

Radiation therapy for some head and neck cancers may involve the irradiation of hypothalamus, pituitary gland, or the thyroid gland. Endocrine abnormalities may be evident clinically when dose to these glands exceeds 40 Gy and >75 % of the gland is exposed to irradiation [20].

11   Laryngeal Edema

Edema of the arytenoids may occur following laryngeal irradiation [20]. Conservative management of laryngeal edema includes voice rest, the use of antibiotics for ulceration, and possibly steroids. Persistence of edema longer than 3 months after radiotherapy completion is indicative of recurrent or persistent tumor. Laryngectomy may be needed for management of laryngeal edema for these patients [20].

12   Dysphagia

Dysphagia may present as an evident symptom in patients receiving radiotherapy to the head and neck region. Underlying factors may include direct toxicity to taste buds, xerostomia, infections, and physiologic conditioning [19]. More than 30 Gy total dose of fractionated irradiation may result in reduced acuity of sweet, sour, bitter, and salt tastes [19]. Loss of taste sensation has been attributed to damage to the microvilli and outer surface of the taste cells. Although permanent hypogeusia may develop in some patients, taste acuity usually returns 2–3 months after radiotherapy completion. The use of zinc supplementation has been recommended for prevention of radiation-induced oropharyngeal mucositis and oral discomfort [21].

Loss of appetite may occur in cancer patients along with dysphagia, mucositis, taste loss, xerostomia, nausea, and vomiting which worsens quality of life due to poor nutritional intake. Oral pain may also prevent some patients from eating. Nutritional counseling may be recommended for keeping the patient aware of nutritional deficiencies and their consequences. The use of nasogastric feeding tubes or percutaneous esophageal gastrostomy may be considered in the presence of significant swallowing impairment. Total parenteral nutrition is usually reserved for patients unable to eat because of mucositis or nausea [19].

13   Pharyngeal Dysfunction

Dysfunction of pharyngeal transport and swallowing has been reported following chemoradiotherapy of head and neck cancers [22–25]. Bolus transport and clearance may be limited in patients with pharyngeal transport dysfunction, and increased risk of aspiration may be observed in the presence of swallowing dysfunction. Sparing pharyngeal constrictor muscles by IMRT may decrease the risk of pharyngeal dysfunction and thus decreasing swallowing problems.

14   Brachial Plexopathy

Brachial plexopathy is an infrequent but debilitating complication of head and neck cancer radiotherapy without efficacious cure [26]. The use of IMRT in the management of head and neck cancers has clearly contributed to normal tissue sparing; however, doses to brachial plexus may be increased with this treatment modality [27]. Symptoms of brachial plexopathy may be underreported in patients receiving radiotherapy for head and neck cancers. 12 % of the patients undergoing radiotherapy for head and neck cancers were reported to suffer from brachial plexus-associated neuropathy in a recent study [28]. Common symptoms of brachial plexus-associated neuropathy included ipsilateral pain, numbness/tingling, motor weakness, and/or muscle atrophy [28]. Of note, a significantly higher proportion of patients suffered from neuropathic symptoms when dose to the brachial plexus exceeded 70 Gy, implicating the presence of a potential threshold effect [28]. Stemming from these concerns, brachial plexus is typically delineated as an organ at risk in current head and neck IMRT applications.

15   Spinal Cord Injury

Symptoms of radiation-induced spinal cord injury called radiation myelitis may show great diversity among the affected patients depending on its severity. Paresthesias including tingling sensation and Lhermitte's sign, numbness, motor weakness, loss of sphincter control, total paraparesis, and paraplegia may occur. Time-dose-fractionation features, irradiated volume, the use of chemical/biologic modifiers such as methotrexate, cisplatin, and etoposide may affect the risk of developing radiation-induced spinal cord injury. Shortening the interval between radiotherapy fractions may reduce the tolerance of spinal cord to irradiation. Decreased intensity on T1-weighted images, increased intensity on T2-weighted images, and cord swelling or atrophy may be detected on MR imaging [29, 30].

16   Temporal Lobe Necrosis (TLN)

Temporal lobe necrosis is a severe late complication usually occurring in patients receiving radiotherapy for nasopharyngeal carcinoma. Since temporal lobes are bilaterally exposed to radiation in nasopharyngeal carcinoma radiotherapy, radiation-induced necrosis may develop as a rare but debilitating complication. Symptoms of TLN may include headaches, dizziness, personality changes, impairment of short-term memory, mental confusion, epileptic seizures, and increased intracranial pressure. It may be difficult to distinquish between radiation-induced TLN and recurrent disease. Positron emission tomography, single-photon emission computed tomography, and magnetic spectroscopy may be used for detection of TLN [31]. Steroids, surgical interventions, anticoagulants, anti-platelets, vitamins, hyperbaric oxygen, and bevacizumab may be used in the management of TLN [31].

Other than these aforementioned side effects, radiotherapy of head and neck cancers may result in adverse effects in cornea, lacrimal gland, lens, retina, and optic tract. Radiation-induced cataract may be treated with surgery. Lubrication, patching, and antibiotic drops may be used in the management of keratitis and dry eyes.

References

1. Beyzadeoglu M, Ozyigit G, Ebruli C (2010) Basic radiation oncology, 1st edn. Springer, Berlin
2. Bergonie J, Tribondeau L (1906) Interprétation de quelques résultats de la radiothérapie et essaide fixation d'une technique rationelle. CR Acad Sci 143:983–985
3. Koga DH, Salvajoli JV, Alves FA (2008) Dental extractions and radiotherapy in head and neck oncology: review of the literature. Oral Dis 14:40–44
4. Sulaiman F, Huryn JM, Zlotolow IM (2003) Dental extractions in the irradiated head and neck patient: a retrospective analysis of Memorial Sloan-Kettering Cancer Center protocols, criteria, and end results. J Oral Maxillofac Surg 61:1123–1131
5. Eisbruch A, Ten-Haken RK, Kim HM et al (1999) Dose, volume, and function relationships in parotid salivary glands following conformal and intensity-modulated irradiation of head and neck cancer. Int J Radiat Oncol Biol Phys 45:577–587

6. Deasy JO, Moiseenko V, Marks L et al (2010) Radiotherapy dose-volume effects on salivary gland function. Int J Radiat Oncol Biol Phys 76(3 Suppl):S58–63
7. Sood AJ, Fox NF, O'Connell BP et al (2014) Salivary gland transfer to prevent radiation-induced xerostomia: a systematic review and meta-analysis. Oral Oncol 50:77–83
8. Jha N, Harris J, Seikaly H et al (2012) A phase II study of submandibular gland transfer prior to radiation for prevention of radiation-induced xerostomia in head-and-neck cancer (RTOG 0244). Int J Radiat Oncol Biol Phys 84:437–442
9. Jha N, Seikaly H, Harris J et al (2003) Prevention of radiation induced xerostomia by surgical transfer of submandibular salivary gland into submental space. Radiother Oncol 66:283–289
10. Meng Z, Garcia MK, Hu C et al (2012) Randomized controlled trial of acupuncture for prevention of radiation-induced xerostomia among patients with nasopharyngeal carcinoma. Cancer 111:3337–3344
11. Braga FP, Lemos Junior CA, Alves FA et al (2011) Acupuncture for the prevention of radiation-induced xerostomia in patients with head and neck cancer. Braz Oral Res 25:180–185
12. Gu J, Zhu S, Li X et al (2014) Effect of amifostine in head and neck cancer patients treated with radiotherapy: a systematic review and meta-analysis based on randomized controlled trials. PLoS One 9:e95968
13. Hensley ML, Hagerty KL, Kewalramani T et al (2009) American Society of Clinical Oncology 2008 clinical practice guideline update: use of chemotherapy and radiation therapy protectants. J Clin Oncol 27:127–145
14. Rudat V, Münter M, Rades D et al (2008) The effect of amifostine or IMRT to preserve parotid function after radiotherapy of the head and neck region measured by quantitative salivary gland scintigraphy. Radiother Oncol 89:71–80
15. Brizel DM, Wasserman TH, Henke M et al (2000) Phase III randomized trial of amifostine as a radioprotector in head and neck cancer. J Clin Oncol 18:3339–3345
16. Lovelace TL, Fox NF, Sood AJ et al (2014) Management of radiotherapy-induced salivary hypofunction and consequent xerostomia in patients with oral or head and neck cancer: meta-analysis and literature review. Oral Surg Oral Med Oral Pathol Oral Radiol 117:595–607
17. Pimentel MJ, Filho MM, Araújo M et al (2014) Evaluation of radioprotective effect of pilocarpine ingestion on salivary glands. Anticancer Res 34:1993–1999
18. Johnson JT, Ferretti GA, Nethery WJ et al (1993) Oral pilocarpine for post-irradiation xerostomia in patients with head and neck cancer. N Engl J Med 329:390–395
19. Blanco AI, Chao C (2006) Management of radiation-induced head and neck injury. In: Small W Jr, Woloschak GE (eds) Radiation toxicity: a practical guide. Springer Science Media Business, Inc, New York, pp 23–41. ISBN 1-4020-8053-0
20. Fein DA, Coia LR (1996) Head and neck cancer. In: Coia LR, Moylan DJ (eds) Introduction to clinical radiation oncology, 3rd edn. Medical Physics Publishing, Madison, pp 79–121
21. Ertekin MV, Koc M, Karslioglu I et al (2004) Zinc sulfate in the prevention of radiation-induced oropharyngeal mucositis: a prospective, placebo-controlled, randomized study. Int J Radiat Oncol Biol Phys 58:167–174
22. Agarwal J, Palwe V, Dutta D et al (2011) Objective assessment of swallowing function after definitive concurrent (chemo)radiotherapy in patients with head and neck cancer. Dysphagia 26:399–406
23. Forastiere AA, Goepfert H, Maor M et al (2003) Concurrent chemotherapy and radiotherapy for organ preservation in advanced laryngeal cancer. N Engl J Med 349:2091–2098
24. Eisbruch A, Lyden T, Bradford CR et al (2002) Objective assessment of swallowing dysfunction and aspiration after radiation concurrent with chemotherapy for head-and-neck cancer. Int J Radiat Oncol Biol Phys 53:23–28
25. Kotz T, Abraham S, Beitlcr JJ et al (1999) Pharyngeal transport dysfunction consequent to an organ-sparing protocol. Arch Otolaryngol Head Neck Surg 125:410–413
26. Schierle C, Winograd JM (2004) Radiation-induced brachial plexopathy: review. Complication without a cure. J Reconstr Microsurg 20:149–152
27. Chen AM, Hall WH, Li BQ et al (2011) Intensity-modulated radiotherapy increases dose to brachial plexus compared with conventional radiotherapy for head and neck cancer. Br J Radiol 84:58–63

28. Chen AM, Hall WH, Li J et al (2012) Brachial plexus-associated neuropathy after high-dose radiation therapy for head-and-neck cancer. Int J Radiat Oncol Biol Phys 84:165–169
29. Koehler PJ, Verbiest H, Jager J et al (1996) Delayed radiation myelopathy: serial MR-imaging and pathology. Clin Neurol Neurosurg 98:197–201
30. Wang PY, Shen WC, Jan JS (1992) Magnetic resonance imaging in radiation myelopathy. Am J Neuroradiol 13:1049–1055
31. Chen J, Dassarath M, Yin Z et al (2011) Radiation induced temporal lobe necrosis in patients with nasopharyngeal carcinoma: a review of new avenues in its management. Radiat Oncol 6:128

Index

© Springer International Publishing Switzerland 2015
M. Beyzadeoglu et al. (eds.), *Radiation Therapy for Head and Neck Cancers:
A Case-Based Review*, DOI 10.1007/978-3-319-10413-3

Printing: Ten Brink, Meppel, The Netherlands
Binding: Stürtz, Würzburg, Germany